POST–WAR MOTHERS

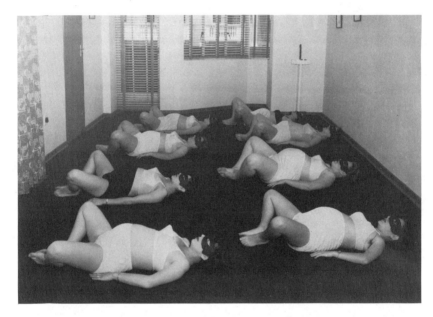

Women in an ante-natal class exercising. Illustration from Dick-Read's book *Antenatal Illustrated*, 1955. Courtesy of the Wellcome Institute Library, London.

POST-WAR MOTHERS

Childbirth Letters to Grantly Dick-Read,
1946–1956

Edited with an Introduction by

Mary Thomas

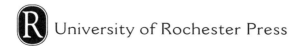 University of Rochester Press

First published 1997

University of Rochester Press
668 Mt. Hope Avenue
Rochester, NY 14620   USA

and at P.O. Box 9
Woodbridge, Suffolk IP12 3DF
United Kingdom

ISBN 1–878822–87–X

Library of Congress Cataloging-in-Publication Data

    Post-war mothers : childbirth letters to Grantly Dick-Read, 1946–1956
      / edited with an introduction by Mary Thomas.
         p.   cm.
     Includes bibliographical references.
     ISBN 1–878822–87–X (alk. paper)
     1. Dick-Read, Grantly, 1890–1959—Correspondence.
     2. Obstetricians—Correspondence.   3. Mothers—Correspondence.
     4. Natural childbirth—Correspondence.   I. Thomas, Mary, 1950 June
     6–
     RG661.D55P67   1997
     618.4´5—dc21   97–42313
                                                       CIP

British Library Cataloguing-in-Publication Data
A catalogue record for this book is
available from the British Library

Designed and typeset by Cornerstone Composition Services
Printed in the United States of America
This publication is printed on acid-free paper

Contents

Contents   vii

Preface

*I*n the aftermath of World War II, women in the United States and Britain were expected to embrace the role of wife, mother, and caretaker of the family. Yet, during World War II, it was not uncommon for women to be employed outside of the home. They were needed to keep the war-time economies going by producing war-time supplies and contributing to the war effort. Upon the conclusion of the war, public sphere roles for Anglo-US women were re-evaluated. This re-evaluation did not lead to a public debate of women's roles; instead, the shift occurred by eliminating them from the workplace. The prevailing opinion was that men must have the right to return to their jobs and resume their roles as wage earner in the family upon their return from World War II. Both Britain and the United States made it clear that men could expect to resume their jobs and/or have priority in the hiring for new jobs. Women workers were made to feel that they had always been considered temporary workers. By being told this, they were being told outright that they were expendable laborers in the public sphere.

Some women wanted to return to the private sphere, and others did not. Nonetheless, the point is that decisions were made for women based on the needs of the post-war British and United States economies and the men returning from war. These decisions had the effect of establishing the traditional family as the norm in post-war US and British societies. This traditional family had clear expectations for women in the private sphere while advocating roles for men in the public sphere. Both the United States and Britain wanted, indeed, expected women to be homemakers and rearers of children. The emphasis of this study is not on the women who found their way back into the job markets when the economies changed from a wartime to consumer focus. Instead, the emphasis is on the private sphere expectations for women in the post-war United States and Britain.

A major area in which these private sphere expectations can be seen was in the process of childbirth. Specifically, the trend in Britain and the United States shifted from home birth to hospital (scientific) delivery with obstetricians (mostly male at the time) in total control. In this setting, the drugged and/or anesthetized woman had almost no say in her delivery; her conscious participation was minimal at best, and as the letters reveal, often unwelcome.

The appearance of Grantly Dick-Read's book on natural childbirth, *Revelation of Childbirth* published in London in 1942, and published with the title *Childbirth Without Fear* in the United States in 1944 marked a turning point. Grantly Dick-Read, a British obstetrician, was the first to advocate childbirth without anaesthetics in his book, *Natural Childbirth*, published in England in 1933. Dick-Read's books made available to women the method he had been using in his London practice for some years. His emphasis on educating women about childbirth, on relieving pain through relaxation and breathing, and on demanding women be conscious during the entire birth process was revolutionary in its time, and the reception by his colleagues was not enthusiastic. Many women, on the other hand, accepted the principles of the method, but found themselves caught up in conflict. Dick-Read's emphasis on the ability of 95–97% of women being able to give birth painlessly led to feelings of inadequacy among the women who felt pain; they felt they had failed. Another result of the application of Dick-Read's method in post-war society was the conflict many women felt between being granted control over the birth process and a similar control being taken away in their role in the public sector, as many forfeited their jobs to returning veterans.

The Letters

Over the years, Grantly Dick-Read received thousands of letters from women all over the world. Approximately 3,400 letters, dating from 1933 until Dick-Read's death in 1959, are part of the collection of his private and professional papers kept in the Contemporary Medical Archives Centre at the Wellcome Institute for the History of Medicine in London. Most of the letters are accompanied by copies of Dick-Read's reply; many have follow-up letters from the women. The twenty-six years of correspondence is a unique view of women's experiences of childbirth told in their own words, and the collection is also a chronicle of Dick-Read's career. For this volume the letters were specifically chosen with the women's experiences in mind. Much of the correspondence contains what could be typically referred to as "fan mail." A great many letters are also repetitive in their request for the names and addresses of doctors in their areas who practiced Dick-Read's methods for childbirth.

The sixty-four letters presented in this volume are representative of the collection as a whole. These letters form a chorus of the eloquent voices of women, reflecting their joys, sorrows, questions, and deep feelings of concern for themselves. The overriding criteria in choosing the sixty-four letters was that the voices of the women be heard. A second consideration was that the patient/physician relationship in post-war Britain and the United States be documented through the correspondence. Finally, a third factor that played a role was an attempt to illustrate that Grantly Dick-Read and his writings on natural childbirth represent a turning point in the history of childbirth. The time period of the letters, 1946–1956, was not a conscious limitation placed on the research, but rather something that just happened during the editing process.

Overwhelmingly, the letters in the whole collection appear to be from middle-class women. The letters from women in the United States are approximately 18% of the entire collection. Of that figure 36% were from women in the Eastern United States, 21% from the Midwest, 21% from the Southern states, and approximately 22% from the West. The letters from Britain represent 59% of the collection distributed as follows: 18% from central London; 49% from Southeast England; 33% from the rest of England; and the remaining 2% from Scotland, Wales, and Ireland.*

Because of the strict regulations by the Wellcome Institute for maintaining confidentiality, all names have been omitted. Where the author of the letter referred to the name of a child, I changed it to read "Baby G" for a girl and "Infant B" for a boy.** I took great pains to maintain the anonymity of the authors of the letters; this was done by omitting names of family, friends, physicians, nurses, hospitals, street addresses, and anything else I considered potentially revealing.

---

*   I sincerely thank John Davison for sorting through my notes on the towns of England and helping me to arrive at this geographic distribution.

**   I wish to thank Maura Hametz for suggesting this form of identification for the children.

Acknowledgments

*I*n the final research phase of my doctoral dissertation I attempted to locate the papers of Dr. John Bowlby, the prominent post-war British child psychiatrist. When I inquired about the papers at the Contemporary Medical Archives Centre in the Library of the Wellcome Institue for the History of Medicine, London, I was referred to Lesley A. Hall, Senior Assistant Archivist. She informed me that the Bowlby papers were in the process of being catalogued and unavailable for research. However, she went on to ask what I was working on and how I was using Bowlby's work. When I completed my, hopefully concise, explanation of "The Politics of Childhood in Post-War Britain," Lesley suggested that I might be interested in the doctor who pioneered natural childbirth, Dr. Grantly Dick-Read. My initial reaction was that I probably would not have need for this archival material. But I was there and hoped that by spending some time with the Dick-Read papers it would not be problematic for me to work with the Bowlby papers when they became available. On 22 March 1994, I ordered my first box of the letters exchanged between Grantly Dick-Read and women in post-war Britain and was immediately convinced of the historical importance of the women's stories. I offer my first and very warm "thank you" to Lesley for her professional interest in this project. She offered exceptional advice through the many stages that a research project takes to its final point of publication. As I bring this project to its conclusion she is more than a valued colleague she is a good friend as well.

My second "thank you" is extended to my three teachers, James Cronin, Peter Weiler, and Larry Wolff, for directing the program in which I grew from a graduate student into a scholar. At the early stages of this project, James Cronin offered solid advice on research and important encouragement for my idea for an edited volume of letters. It was Peter Weiler who suggested that I go to the National Register of Archives and try to find the papers of John Bowlby—and while looking for one thing I found another. Peter offered scholarly support for this project, read the first version of the manuscript and gave intelligent and valuable criticism. Moreover, his paitent, good advice and guidance as I sought a publisher was extremely helpful. My thoughts on twentieth-century epistolary discourse greatly benefited from Larry Wolff's publications analyzing the eighteenth-century letters of Maria Theresa, Marie Antoinnette and Madame de Sevigne and his enthusiasm for my idea helped to finish the project on a positive level. They always asked me for the same high standards of scholarship they ask of themselves, and I am sincerely appreciative.

It has been a distinct pleasure working with the University of Rochester Press. I offer a special "thank you" to Sean M. Culhane for believing in this project and my vision for the way the research should be presented. Louise Goldberg has been a patient and excellent editor, and I have enjoyed working with her by phone and mail. I also thank Professor Jean Pedersen of the Eastman School of Music, University of Rochester, who reviewed the original manuscript and offered substantial, compelling, and intelligent suggestions for its many revisions.

Grantly Dick-Read's children, Diana Dick-Read Nicholson, John Dick-Read and Robert Dick-Read, have been very supportive of this project. They have relived their childhoods with me, and, for their personal insights on their father, I am deeply grateful. Diana and her husband, Alistair Nicholson, gave a lovely lunch in their home with John and Robert for my husband and me. I remember with much fondness sitting around the table after lunch talking about "the family" with Diana, John, and Robert. I am especially grateful to John for giving me many family letters and photographs to add to his father's private and professional papers at the Wellcome Institute. Their friendship has been a special bonus from working on this project.

Working in the Poynter Room in the Library of the Wellcome Institute for the History of Medicine is a privilege and a pleasure. I always looked forward to going to work because of the professional, intelligent, and efficient staff. I would like to thank everyone who helped me and answered my many questions: Julia Sheppard, Shirley Dixon, Jennifer Haynes, Isobel Hunter, Sara Bakewell; and to Jason Conduct, who retrieved my boxes of documents upon request. I regret that I cannot name all the others personally.

My sincere thanks goes to Maura Hametz for her encouragement and enthusiasm for this project and the many conversations we had on women in the post-war period. She extensively edited the first version of this manuscript and recommended that I create a thematic table of contents for the letters. Maura was eager to do more and had there been time she would have, again, edited Part I. I am grateful to the many who listened to and read at different times various versions of my work on Grantly Dick-Read and offered excellent comments: Rima Apple, Donald Caton, Jennifer Haynes, Irvine Loudon, Hilary Marland, John Macnicol, Joyce Malcolm, Lara Marks, Julia Sheppard, Jillian Strang, Susan Tananbaum, and Susan Williams.

Although many have helped me by editing my various versions of the manuscript, listening to my ideas, and/or offering suggestions, I accept full responsibility for the end result and know that it would have benefited further, had I incorporated more of their suggestions.

The many trips to London to research this project were made all the more pleasant because Harriet and John Davison included my husband and me in their family Sunday dinners. Their family, Mrs. Sharlie Davison, Sarah, Christopher, Victoria Riding, and Jack welcomed us and were very patient with my "childbirth stories." I have greatly benefited from Sharlie's rememberances of Thea Cannon Dick-Read. I sincerely thank them, with love, for their interest in my work and the many warm, good times.

My friends contributed to the various stages of this project by remaining interested, enthusiastic, and supportive: Jane Graham and Kevin Dwyer, Gerri and Frank Sullivan, Pat and Tom McInerney, and Cynthia Hartshorn.

Over the years I have enjoyed great support and love from Shannon Thomas, who was in London when I first discovered the letters at the Wellcome Institute. Claudia Thomas Backes and Glenn Backes have been unfailing in their belief in my abilities, and I am grateful for their love. My life is all the better because the three of them are a part of it.

Claude Thomas, my husband, is the most important source of love, intelligence, and support in my life. It was his idea for me to return to college as an undergraduate after being out of school for twelve years. He was the first to encourage me to go further and attend graduate school for a Master's and then the Ph.D., and he loved me all along the long road of my education with the consequent changes. He read, listened to, and commented on every version of this project. I have known no greater love than his, and I have not reaped so many rewards from one piece of advice—"Go back to school and put your intelligence to work." I love him. I thank him. For all that he is to me, this book is dedicated to him.

Chronology of
Grantly Dick-Read's Life

26 January 1890	Birth of Grantly Dick Read to Robert John Read and Fanny Maria
	Education: Bishop's Stortford College St. John's College, Cambridge University London Hospital
1914	Receives degree from Cambridge University and joins Royal Army Medical Corps at outbreak of World War I
1918	Cambridge University, Demonstrator in Pathology
1919	London Hospital, resident staff
1920	Writes first book on natural childbirth (unpublished)
	Receives MD (Cambridge) for thesis on "Bacteriology on Malignant Endocarditis"
1921	Marries Dorothea (Thea) Cannon
1923	Establishes private practice partnership in Woking
1923–1948	Practices in Woking and Harley Street
1926	Complaint to General Medical Council that the practice was advertising
1933	*Natural Childbirth* published by Heinemann; Dick-Read contributed to the cost of publication
1934	Working partnership dissolved. Dick-Read established a practice at the same location on his own
1942	Publication of *Revelation* of Childbirth (1944 *Childbirth Without Fear* in the United States)
1943	Publication of *Motherhood in the Postwar World*
1947	Tours the United States lecturing on natural childbirth
	Publication of *Birth of a Child*
1948–1953	Relocates and resides in South Africa to practice medicine

1949	Lawsuit against the South African Medical and Dental Council over their refusal to register him
1950	Publication of *Introduction to Motherhood*
1952	Obtains divorce from first wife, Dorothea, after 31 years of marriage and four children; marries Jessica Bennett and adopts her two sons from her first marriage
1953	Films four women in childbirth before his departure from South Africa
	Safari with Jessica and the two sons to witness childbirth among native African women
1954	Returns and reestablishes a home in England; retires from practice; concentrates on publishing, correspondence, and lectures
1955	Publication of *Antenatal Illustrated*
1956	Publication of *No Time for Fear*
	Papal Encyclical on the moral and spiritual validity of natural childbirth teachings
	Film, *Childbirth Without Fear*, released
	Argo Records releases long playing record, *Childbirth Without Fear*, which recorded a labor conducted on Dick-Read's principles of natural childbirth
	Dick-Read granted an audience by the Pope and presented with the Silver Papal Medal
1957	Excepts from film shown on BBC television
	Publication of biography, *Doctor Courageous*, by A. Noyes Thomas
1957–1958	Engages in an extensive lecture tour of the United States and Canada
1958	Officially legalizes the hyphenation of his name
11 June 1959	Dies in Norfolk, England

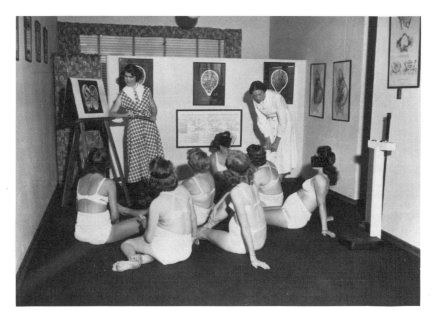

Women in an ante-natal class. Illustration from Dick-Read's book *Antenatal Illustrated*, 1955. Courtesy of the Wellcome Institute Library, London.

Part 1

Grantly Dick-Read and Natural Childbirth:
A Turning Point in the History of Childbirth

Grantly Dick-Read and Natural Childbirth: A Turning Point in the History of Childbirth

Background: Childbirth in Britain and the United States

At the end of the seventeenth century childbirth was a social occasion, a woman-centered and woman-controlled event that took place in the home. Women delivered women, helping each other in an event that was unique to women. Upon learning of an impending birth, a woman gathered around her a group of trusted and "experienced" women to be present for the delivery of her child. This trusted group offered her moral support. Further, the group insured that she had company and was not left alone at any point during the labor. As well as women for company, there would very likely be a midwife in attendance or the woman who was locally known as having years of experience delivering other women in the community. The midwife did the actual delivering of the baby and the chores associated with administering to the immediate needs of the mother and infant. When the midwife was confronted with complications that were outside her realm of abilities, she called in a surgeon. If a surgeon was called in, it meant that either the mother or the infant (or both) were dying. The anticipation of excruciating pain and the fear of death in childbirth were the realities of being pregnant. And being pregnant was very much a part of a married woman's life.

The male physician began taking an active role in delivering babies in the eighteenth century. The use of instruments, particularly forceps, was the domain of the male physician. In the United States by the eighteenth century, an attending midwife became less common with the increasing role of the physician. However, in Britain, the role of the midwife continued as an important option for women in labor. As physicians began to assume the role of delivering women they simulta-neously challenged midwives' lack of credentials. This challenge, instead of eliminating the midwives in Britain, required them to become licensed to carry on their work delivering babies.

If instrument births served as the entrance for males into the routine delivering of babies in the eighteenth century, it was the use of drugs in the nineteenth century that solidified their place of prominence in this formerly female-centered event. The control of childbirth by the women who were delivering and the women who were administering to the mothers and infants declined with advances in medicine. The advance of scientific childbirth enabled physicians, and ultimately hospitals, to secure a permanent role in the need for women to have their babies delivered professionally and in institutions.

Although men were moving into the arena of delivering women of their babies, it was not until late in the nineteenth century that it be-came an "acceptable" medical specialty for men. Again, the midwife in Britain continued to be an option while in the United States, by the end of the nineteenth century, there was a concerted effort on the part of the medical community to eliminate midwives completely. This was effective by the beginning of the twentieth century.

While the nineteenth century continued to see the majority of women having their babies at home, the major advance in the history of childbirth in the nineteenth century was the use of anesthetics such as ether and chloroform. The advent of chloroform was seen as a ma-jor breakthrough in aiding women through the extreme difficulties and pain of birth. With the belief that drugs would play a role in limiting pain, women felt that something had genuinely been done to help their plight in childbirth. There were, however, drawbacks to the use of an-esthetics. They did not fully eliminate pain in childbirth because they could not be used until very late in labor. There was also fear of the anesthetic's impact on the physiological functions of the muscles needed in childbirth as well as the consequence that the use of any kind of drugs would have on the infant. The after-effects of ether and/or chlo-roform were also very unpleasant, as women attest to in some of the post-war letters that follow in Part 2.

Scopolamine was the drug that heightened expectations for the per-fect birth in the twentieth century. This drug, developed in Germany in 1902 and most commonly used beginning around 1914, was associ-ated with "twilight sleep." Scopolamine blocked the experience of labor and birth from the woman's memory. Given by injection at the onset of labor, it produced an amnesiac state. A pain killer was given in conjunc-tion with it; the woman was relaxed and made unaware of her physical condition and her immediate surroundings. Once the drug worked through the woman's system, she woke up oblivious to the birth of her infant. One of the advantages of scopolamine was that it could be administered at any point during labor, as it did not affect the body physiologically. From this standpoint the patient and the physician saw scopolamine as a beneficial drug in childbirth. As stated above, women's memories of childbirth were eliminated while their muscles and internal organs were going through the physical exercise of delivering the baby. Therefore, it was not uncommon for women during their drugged stupor to scream and writhe in physical pain while their memories blocked any recall of the physical discomfort. The use of scopolamine required the hospitalization of the woman in childbirth, as it necessitated administration by a physician.

A further impact of drugs was how women viewed childbirth and themselves in childbirth. With the introduction of drugs and the resulting requirement for hospitalization, women distanced, even absented, themselves both from the childbirth experience and from their bodies. Emily Martin has written about the alienation of women from their bodies in childbirth.[1] She suggests in her work that women came to view what was happening to their bodies as an involuntary experience. The women lost control of what was happening to their bodies in childbirth and became dependent upon their organs to act independently. This is consistent with scientific childbirth which depends on women being ignorant of what is happening during labor and embracing drugs. In the letters that follow, women felt removed from the childbirth experience, and consequently, in the process, a loneliness engulfed them.

Making childbirth a medical event is at the heart of Judith Walzer Leavitt's book, *Brought to Bed: Childbearing in America, 1750–1950*. Leavitt details the transformation of childbirth from a home-centered, woman-controlled experience to a hospital-centered, physician-controlled medical event. Further, Leavitt constructs women's role in this transformation by explaining that women participated in it as a means of making the childbirth experience safer and less painful. Clearly the introduction of drugs was an attempt to help women. But the consequence was that physicians and hospitals took control of this event and told women how they felt, what they needed, and how (in some instances even when) the delivery would take place. There are letters in

---

[1]   Emily Martin, *The Woman in the Body: A Cultural Analysis of Reproduction* (Boston: Beacon Press, 1987).

Part 2 that show the physician's control sometimes took place even though the patient objected.

Leavitt writes: "The twilight-sleep movement helped change the definition of birth from a natural home event, as it was in the nineteenth century, to an illness requiring hospitalization and physician attendance."[2] A key concept here is alluded to by the term "illness"; childbirth was seen by many physicians as something not at all natural, in fact, pathologic. Because twilight sleep required so much professional management by doctors and nurses, and because of the often unpredictable reactions of many women, it was short-lived as a method for giving birth. However, it helped spearhead the total control of the childbirth experience by professionals and institutions, and made the use of drugs, instruments, and a prevalence toward Cesarean sections more acceptable by the 1940s. Total management of childbirth outside the hands of pregnant women was completed by the 1950s. Specifically, in the United States by 1950, 88% of all births were in the hospital, and in the 1960s and 1970s delivering babies outside the sterile, managed delivery room of a hospital was considered dangerous and foolish and was practically nonexistent.[3] In Britain, 66% of births in the late 1950s took place in institutions, and by 1974 that figure jumped to 96% of all births taking place in institutions.[4]

One of the significant aspects of Irvine Loudon's study, *Death in Childbirth: An International Study of Maternal Care and Maternal Mortality, 1800–1950*, is his analysis of the way women were treated once giving birth was removed from the homes and placed in the hospitals of Britain and the United States. Loudon suggests that where women gave birth (provided there were no complications) did not matter as much as how they were treated. In other words, the treatment by the caregivers toward pregnant women and/or women in labor was more crucial in the overall quality of the experience of delivery than the immediate physical surroundings.[5] The evidence contained in the correspondence that follows confirms Loudon's assertion for both the British and US childbirth experiences in the post-war period.

In *The American Way of Birth*, Jessica Mitford states that it was predominantly wealthy American women with the means to travel abroad

---

[2]   Judith Walzer Leavitt, *Brought to Bed: Childbearing in America, 1750–1950* (Oxford: Oxford University Press, 1986), 140–41.

[3]   Ibid., 171.

[4]   Ann Oakely, *Women Confined: Towards a Sociology of Childbirth* (New York: Schocken Books, 1980), 121.

[5]   Irvine Loudon. *Death in Childbirth: An International Study of Maternal Care and Maternal Mortality, 1800–1950* (Oxford: Oxford University Press, 1992).

who were trying twilight sleep and the Dick-Read method of natural childbirth and later the method of Lamaze.[6] In fact the letters that follow in Part 2 will dispute what Mitford writes. These letters clearly indicate that women in the United States read the Dick-Read antenatal advice books and in many cases attempted to go it alone—with or without the advice of their obstetricians. Further, Margarete Sandelowski asserts in her conclusion to *Pain, Pleasure, and American Childbirth: From the Twilight Sleep to the Read Method, 1914–1960*, that the natural childbirth movement was not a contest between women and their physicians. She states:

> Natural Childbirth, in the 1940s and 1950s, was distinctively nonfeminist, if not antifeminist, and promedical in control of the childbirth arena. It is simply inaccurate to politicize the early Natural Childbirth movement by depicting women and physicians as adversaries on two sides of the Natural Childbirth argument.[7]

The letters that follow in Part 2 question Sandelowski's conclusion. There are letters detailing the struggle that women had in the United States to find a physician to participate in the natural childbirth experience. As some of the letters show, doctors frequently acquiesced, only to assert control by administering drugs against the wishes of the laboring woman.

In her "Bibliographical Essay," Sandelowski states that the three major participants in the US natural childbirth dialogue were physicians, nurses, and childbearing women. However, while seeking out the literature of the doctors and nurses, she did not interview women who had given birth, because she believed that oral accounts of past childbirth experiences would be influenced by the current childbirth debates. Sandelowski futher comments:

> The group who emerges as the least articulate is childbearing women who left few firsthand accounts of their views and experiences. Attempts were made to obtain materials such as unpublished 'letters to the editor' of popular magazines, women's responses on evaluation questionnaires given them during their hospital stay, and other personal documents, but these were not available. Many of these items were discarded long ago, and women were simply less likely to record their personal experiences in childbirth than professionals were to record their clinical experiences and professional beliefs.[8]

---

[6]   Jessica Mitford, *The American Way of Birth* (New York: Dutton, 1992), 63.
[7]   Margarete Sandelowski, *Pain, Pleasure, and American Childbirth: From the Twilight Sleep to the Read Method, 1914-1960* (Westport, Ct.: Greenwood Press, 1984), 136.
[8]   Ibid., 139.

This volume of edited letters from women documenting their child-birth experiences shows Sandelowski's work would have benefited from their stories. The Dick-Read papers became available for scholarly research in 1985, one year after Sandelowski's book, but, nonetheless, they did exist at the Wellcome Institute for the History of Medicine in London, and provide a powerful voice to the history of childbirth.

In the history of childbirth the twentieth century ushered in the transference of the event from the domestic confines of the home, with pregnant women being delivered by a birth attendant that best suited their needs, to the confines of an institution. When childbirth became a hospital-centered event, women lost their voice in where and how they gave birth. What in earlier centuries was under the control of women fell, by the middle of the twentieth century, under the control of doctors and institutions.

Grantly Dick-Read

In his works on natural childbirth (especially *Revelation of Childbirth* and *Childbirth Without Fear*), Dick-Read introduced the concept that relaxation at the onset of labor was the most effective means of experiencing a conscious, joyful childbirth in 95%–97% of cases. He wrote that informing and educating women on what was happening to their bodies during pregnancy and labor would enable them to relax. Relaxation, he maintained, would eliminate fear and the tension brought on by lack of knowledge. In his antenatal literature, he concluded that if a woman felt pain it would not be significant enough to require drugs.

Dick-Read believed that one of the advantages of natural childbirth was women's overwhelming joy in giving birth. In April 1954, he was Guest of the Week on the BBC's Woman's Hour. During this broadcast he spoke of joyful childbirth:

> Thousands of women from all countries of the world have testified to the merits of this preparation [i.e., natural childbirth] for motherhood. They are no longer afraid but want more babies as soon as possible. Any discomfort they may have had was too slight to justify in their minds unconsciousness when the babe was born. There was no interference by the medical attendant and the joy of watching the birth of the child, hearing its first cry and holding it in their arms immediately after it was separated from them was too wonderful to be missed and remained a bond of happiness between the mother and child for all time.[9]

---

[9] Grantly Dick-Read papers in the Contemporary Medical Archives Centre at the Wellcome Institute for the History of Medicine, CMAC: PP/GDR/G.28, "Radio and TV Broadcasts: Correspondence, Transcripts, 1954–1958," 28 April 1954.

Dick-Read's best examples of natural childbirth were working-class women and native African women. His first model for natural childbirth was a working-class woman from Whitechapel he attended as a medical student at London Hospital in 1911. Less than a year after his arrival at London Hospital he began administering to the sick in some of the poorest areas of London. On one such visit he entered a small, damp, poorly lit room in Whitechapel, and delivered a woman of her first child. He recounted this event in his unpublished autobiography:

> As the baby's head made its appearance at the outlet of the birth canal and the dilatation of the passage was at a stage where I felt there should be discomfort and pain, I tried to persuade my patient to let me put the mask over her face so that she could inhale some chloroform. But the girl refused the mask, saying that she had no need of this help.[10]

Later as he prepared to leave, he asked the woman why she refused assistance and she responded: "It didn't hurt. It wasn't meant to, was it Doctor?"[11] This became his favorite story. Further, it was a turning point for how he shaped his medical career and ultimately influenced women around the world while remaining a physician on the fringe of his profession.

Grantly Dick-Read (his middle and last name were legally hyphenated in 1958) was born in Beccles, Suffolk, England, in 1890. He earned his MD from Cambridge University in 1920 after serving in the Royal Army Medical Corps during World War I. While serving in Gallipoli, he was badly injured and after recuperation served out the war in France. During his service in World War I, surrounded by maimed soldiers and death, Dick-Read spent a great amount of his time and concentration perfecting his theories of pain and committed himself to a future in obstetrics.

Dick-Read spent a short time in private practice in Eastbourne, Hampshire, before moving his practice in 1923 to Woking, Surrey, with consulting rooms in Harley Street, London. He married Dorothea (Thea) Cannon in 1921, and they had two sons and two daughters. Thea did not support his career and his teachings on natural childbirth. He felt isolated both at home and among his peers who did not fully accept his ideas. Dick-Read wanted to become a member of the Royal College of Obstetricians and Gynaecologists. However, he refused to sit for the required examination, because he felt he had already proven

---

[10] Grantly Dick-Read papers in the Contemporary Medical Archives Centre, Wellcome Institute Library, London, PP/GDR/D.92, "Autobiography," Installment Two, 20–21.
[11] Ibid.

himself worthy with his books, publications, lectures, and international prominence. In fact, he was insulted by the suggestion of the
examination.

After World War II, the Royal College offered Dick-Read a building
suitable for delivering pregnant women and teaching his methods of
natural childbirth. At the inspection of the facilities, he only saw a dam-
aged post-war building in an area away from the major London hospitals. He turned down the offer and accused the Royal College of professional jealousy for the rest of his working life.

During World War II, Mrs. Jessica (Jess) Bennett rented a cottage
from the Dick-Read family while her husband was on war duty. She
and her two sons became an extended part of the Dick-Read family.
Jess was an ardent supporter of Dick-Read's methods and work, and
he was convinced that he could not live without this kind of support
any longer. In 1948, before either was divorced, Jessica Bennett and
Grantly Dick-Read set up a home and moved his practice to South Africa. This was a very tumultuous time for him personally and professionally. He left with bitterness toward his peers in England, and with
much sadness and uncertainty over his abandonment of Thea and the
children.

After a lengthy legal battle with the South African government over
his license to practice medicine, Dick-Read attached himself to a hospital on the outskirts of Johannesburg, the Marymount Maternity Hospital, run by Dominican nuns. In 1952, four years after arriving in South
Africa, he obtained a divorce from Thea, and married his second wife,
Jessica Bennett, adopting her two sons.

In 1953, at the age of 64, Dick-Read determined that his work in
South Africa was completed. He, his wife, and two sons set out on a
safari, with the aim of observing non-westernized African women giving birth in their natural environment. At the end of this journey, which
covered 6,000 miles, he was fully satisfied that he had discovered the
truth to childbirth and to life. It was a very simple truth to him, and
more than a discovery it was confirmation of what he had been saying
all along—western civilization was responsible for the destruction of
normal, natural childbirth.

Dick-Read retired from practice on his return to England in 1954.
He spent the remaining years of his life writing, traveling, lecturing,
and engaging in lengthy correspondence with women from around the
world. The correspondence during the last five years of his life reflects
his desire to remain active in his profession. Dick-Read died in 1959 of
complications from a brain hemorrhage, convinced that the Royal College of Obstetricians and Gynaecologists would not recognize his work

because they were jealous of his success. Further, he maintained to the end of his life that only he offered women the means to have babies the way God intended—Natural Childbirth.

Reception of Dick-Read's Method: The Medical Establishment

The medical establishment did not fully accept Dick-Read's natural childbirth theories. He was an anachronism in the practice of medicine. The scientific method of childbirth, which incorporated the use of drugs, instruments, and hospitalization, was at odds with Dick-Read's theories of relaxation, exercise, and proper diet. The idea of being available to a patient in labor for as long as she needed attention was foreign to the obstetricians in the immediate aftermath of World War II. By then they had perfected their specialization, which allowed them to be called in to attend the birth when it was about to happen. They did not spend time coaching their patients, and they were impatient with the women who wanted more of their time than they were willing to allocate. The medical establishment also had difficulty accepting Dick-Read's commingling of medicine and religion. Because he spoke about natural childbirth as God's way for women to have babies, many found reason to dissociate from a physician with ideas they considered old-fashioned and outdated.

The medical professionals in the mid-twentieth century were people of science. Dick-Read challenged the twentieth-century medical profession with eighteenth century and nineteenth-century ideas and colloquy. Dick-Read's ideas put childbirth, in the eyes of his contemporaries, back into the jurisdiction and discourse of religion. Mary Poovey writes that the chloroform debate in the nineteenth century served to distinguish the roles of the clergymen and medical men in the lives of women. The dialogue that the religious men used to subjugate women was adopted by the medical men, but it had the unintended consequence of limiting the power of the medical professionals.[12] When they wrote of the moral or religious implications in this debate, the moral and religious were couched in what was natural. Dick-Read personified this nineteenth-century discourse in the twentieth century when he wrote on natural childbirth. This placed him at odds with his peers in his thinking. Poovey writes that in the mid-nineteenth century the commingling of religious and medical dialogues served to usurp much of the power and professionalization of the medical community over the chlo-

---

[12] Mary Poovey, *Uneven Developments: The Ideological Work of Gender in Mid-Victorian England* (Chicago: University of Chicago Press, 1988).

roform debate. Therefore, what Dick-Read did was to unify the theological with the medical, and this was not viewed as progress by his peers. Dick-Read's ideas did not propel the profession forward; on the contrary, they threatened to turn the clock back. Religion and nature equaled God, while medicine and physiology provided an exercise in controlling women. Consequently, in setting on paper what was normal and natural in childbirth, Dick-Read was able as well to establish what was the normal and natural role for women. This was a very clear throwback to the nineteenth century, when women's roles were defined in society by their biology—their ability to give birth.

Another reason Dick-Read received a lukewarm reception from his peers was that his natural childbirth campaign demanded women's presence in childbirth. This was a direct challenge to the medical profession that had worked very hard to legitimize obstetrics as a specialization. The contested terrain of women's bodies was the attack that Dick-Read launched with his writings and theories of natural childbirth. It threatened the obstetricians' work, as well as the work of the anaesthetists and the profits of the drug companies who depended on the use of certain drugs in childbirth.

What exactly did Dick-Read see as the problem with routinely administering anesthesia and/or analgesia? (I emphasize the routine use of drugs because Dick-Read did not deprive his patients of drugs if they insisted or if complications arose.) His major objection was that by doing so the physician was overstepping his bounds and intruding on nature's work. But more than this, Dick-Read saw obstetric interference as a means of securing a patient for life. In his writings and portrayal of the "average" obstetrician he surely participated in securing a marginal role for himself and his theories among his peers. He states:

> The obstetrician, alas, is in an unenviable position if he has not educated her to understand the experience before it commences, and she is indeed in an unhappy dilemma if the significance of the phenomena of normal labor is not understood by her physician.
>
> If, however, he is not only kind—'perfectly sweet' in fact—but also brilliantly clever (most obstetricians are if they are lucky), at an early stage he can dope her and later administer an anesthetic. It is easier and so much quicker than trying to comprehend the cryptic designs of cruel Nature. The antepenultimate stroke of genius is a forceps extraction, the penultimate dexterity is stitching her perineum, and the ultimate evidence of foresight is a good gynecological patient for years to come, when with advancing of age the obstetric art becomes too exacting.[13]

---

[13] Grantly Dick-Read, *Childbirth Without Fear* (New York: Harper & Brothers, 1953, orig. pub. 1944), 121.

The stereotyping of obstetricians who would not consider natural child-birth or the Dick-Read method for their patients is unmistakable. What was seen by previous generations as advances in childbirth were caus-tically disregarded as tools of the "sweet and clever" in the profession. Writing them off as tools of manipulative obstetricians was, at the very least, a violation of the etiquette of his profession and, at the worst, extreme dogmatic pronouncements.

More was going on in what Dick-Read projected in the above quote, and this clearly helps to account for the tone of the letters that women wrote to him. At this juncture, it would seem appropriate to contem-plate whether or not there was a form of dual manipulation resulting from Dick-Read's monograph on natural childbirth. If a physician made women susceptible to the suggestion that pain was created and con-trolled by the mind, then perhaps women would resist if the physician suggested anesthesia and/or analgesia. As will be seen in the corre-spondence, one consistent theme was that doctors misused anesthesia and/or analgesia, and in some cases forced patients to take them against their will. There will be little question from the letters that some women viewed this as a genuine threat, and felt betrayed by their own obste-tricians. In the end, neither the traditional obstetrician, with his belief in drugged and unconscious birth, nor Dick-Read, with his mission of painless and conscious birth, offered women a choice.

Loudon asserts that the lucrative aspect of childbirth in the United States in the twentieth century was responsible for the slow response accorded to Grantly Dick-Read's theories on natural childbirth. Ob-stetrics, Loudon suggests, presented a steady stream of patients for doctors. I believe there was more. There was a struggle over territory, and, in this case, for obstetricians, women's bodies had become their professional territory. This was a complex issue because as well as chal-lenging the role of physicians in natural childbirth, the role of hospitals was being re-examined as well. Hospitals, and this was particularly so in the United States, had invested in the future of delivering babies by developing specialized hospitals, lying-in hospitals, and, therefore, had as much invested in women "needing" to have their babies in medical institutions as the doctors who built their work around hospital-cen-tered deliveries.

Dick-Read's Method: The Conflict It Established for Women

A significant outcome of Dick-Read's work on natural childbirth was an avalanche of correspondence containing the most intimate details of women's childbirth experiences. On close inspection, the letters reveal poignant accounts of women's lives as told through their experience(s) of childbirth. The strength of the letters that make up the major portion of this volume is that we hear from the women who lived during the immediate aftermath of World War II in the United States and Britain and how they viewed the expectations for their lives through the experience of childbirth. Even more important is what women thought of childbearing and the responsibilities associated with the private sphere.

As will be apparent in the correspondence, Dick-Read's responses to these letters provide a close perspective of his thinking on motherhood and the family, or more specifically, on women's proper role in society in the post-war period. For instance he wrote to a woman in England in 1950:

> I must reply to your letter to assure you that I appreciate you having sent it, for although I do receive many from very widely distributed parts of the world each one comes as a further justification for the principles of physiological childbirth. We have found with the years that it has a much deeper influence than merely enabling a woman to have her babies with the minimum discomfort and greatest possible pleasure, and its influence is showing itself upon society not only in the health of the mothers but in the development of the children. The mother-child relationship, I am sure you will realise, is the basis of a new philosophy, and when man holds in the palm of his hand the power to destroy all living creatures upon the earth there must ultimately come a time when one of two things will happen—either man will be destroyed or by mutual consent of those who are antagonistic in their ideologies destruction will be withheld. Then only one thing will be left—a world with an ideology based upon the philosophy of its purpose and manner of living. To that end the perfection of motherhood is obviously a factor of incalculable importance.[14]

Dick-Read's correspondence with women was a personal extension of his professional publications. By writing at length to women he could reinforce his ideas in an intimate epistolary exchange. Women were caring for themselves by writing candidly about the most personal details of their childbirth experiences. Dick-Read took the opportunity to comment not only on their labors but also on their "pre-ordained" roles in life as evidenced by the above quote. Quite clearly, Dick-Read evoked a powerful, selfish passion from these women that was best expressed through letter writing. But this study shows that letter writing as a means of revealing oneself is not the sole domain of women. As Elizabeth

---

[14]   CMAC: PP/GDR/D.43, "Mothers—United Kingdom, U–Z," 11 April 1950.

Goldsmith writes of the necessity not to stereotype epistolary discourse for seventeenth-century letter writers, the same is so for the twentieth century.[15] The history of a key figure in twentieth-century medicine, Dr. Grantly Dick-Read, takes shape through his letters to women revealing his personal and professional loneliness. The correspondence provides a unique vantage point from which to evaluate his contribution to the history of childbirth.

Dick-Read's antenatal advice books were women's catalyst to initiate a dialogue with him. Ann Oakley writes that she views antenatal advice books as a means of controlling the childbirth experience. Even more than controlling the experience, she sees them as a means of defining the experience. Therefore, because childbirth is a function only women perform, it can be construed that guidelines for how to be a woman are established in this antenatal literature as well. This to Oakely is ironic, since it is a professional and often a man who writes the antenatal advice material. Certainly for the purposes of this study it is the case. Dick-Read, by writing the antenatal advice literature, was, according to Oakley's theories, defining and claiming the birth experience. Oakley states:

> The main vehicle for the programming of women as maternity patients is antenatal advice literature. The evolution of this literature in Britain in fact reflects very closely the chronology of expanding medical jurisdiction over birth.[16]

That women's childbirth literature programmed them as maternity patients can be taken to the next step, in the analysis of Dick-Read's work, by saying that antenatal literature reinforced women's roles and society's expectations for them as traditional mothers. If Dick-Read set some women up to fail in childbirth, then he, too, with his expectations, set even more women up for failure in his expectations of them outside of the act of childbirth.

What Dick-Read's theories meant in terms of women's role in society was very much embedded in his work. An examination of what he wrote privately in correspondence to women in Britain and the United States presents a consistency with his public theories of women's proper roles. For example, he equated womanhood and motherhood to the extent that he believed that giving birth required the same skills that

---

[15] Elizabeth Goldsmith, "Authority, Authenticity, and the Publication of Letters by Women," in *Writing the Female Voice: Essays on Epistolary Literature*, ed. Elizabeth Goldsmith (Boston: Northeastern University Press, 1989), 46–59.

[16] Oakley, *Women Confined*, 34.

women needed in their everyday lives. In 1949 he wrote to a woman in
England having her first baby:

> Remember my three virtues of all good women are required for this [natu-
> ral childbirth]—patience, self-control and the ability to work hard when
> called upon. If you bear those things in mind during labor and, in fact, in
> after life you will have very little to regret.[17]

To a woman in Indiana in 1948, he closed a letter by repeating the same
advice:

> I can do no more than send you my best wishes, and remind you of the
> three great virtues which I preach to those who invite my attentions.
> They are not only applicable in labor, but throughout motherhood—pa-
> tience, self-control and the ability to work hard cheerfully.[18]

His theories directed women toward choosing a delivery without analgesia and anesthesia. He believed that women who were conscious
had joyful deliveries and delivered babies whose personalities would
benefit from mothers who had not been drugged and unconscious.

Ludmilla Jordanova states that the ideas expounded in science and
medicine stand to serve us well in understanding concepts in broader
social contexts.[19] She calls this mediation, and it is with mediation that
we see that medicine, generally, and Grantly Dick-Read, specifically,
served to contribute to a dialogue establishing very definite gender roles
in the post-war period. But he went further than that by stating that
civilized society and middle-class and aristocratic lifestyles had sullied
childbirth. Therefore, for him, learning normal, natural childbirth meant
observing uncivilized people. It is ironic that Dick-Read believed as he
did, because again he was a man out of step with the medical practice
that prevailed in this time period. Clearly, those whom he observed as
the perfect models for natural childbirth were women who were in
charge of their pregnancies and labors, whereas those he believed to be
giving birth in a civilized world were doing so in male-centered and dic-
tated ways. What Grantly Dick-Read did, then, was to attempt to usurp
the power of the uncivilized, women-centered birth procedures and
take charge by writing his antenatal advice and theories. This, then,
was not an attempt to give women power by teaching them natural
childbirth methods but, instead, an opportunity to claim power for himself. What he wrote about natural childbirth from observing working-

---

17 CMAC: PP/GDR/D.13, "English Mothers and Patients Prior to 1950," 4 February 1949.
18 CMAC: PP/GDR/D.106, "Mothers—America—Prior to 1955, H–O," 7 August 1948.
19 Ludmilla Jordanova, *Sexual Visions: Images of Gender in Science and Medicine between the
    Eighteenth and Twentieth Centuries* (Madison, Wisc.: University of Wisconsin Press, 1989).

class women and native African women conforms to Jordanova's concept of mediations by connecting his medical ideas to society beyond the boundaries of science. In other words, in some of the letters that follow, Dick-Read states that women in childbirth must have many of the same qualities necessary for women's roles in everyday life. Therefore, by writing about the childbirth experience within the boundaries of medicine and then taking this ideology into the social context of women's roles in society, Dick-Read is an example of Jordanova's theories of the relevance—and more than relevance—the necessity for scholars to look beyond the immediacy of medical tenets to their broader applications. By examining women's roles through the lens of Jordanova's mediations, a level of control over women's lives is exhibited through the writings of Dick-Read on natural childbirth. But, more can be seen, and that is the control over the definition of what was acceptable and expected of women in the post-war society of England and the United States.

Yet, the natural childbirth techniques offered by Dick-Read required that women be involved. Consequently, when we read the letters that follow, we see that the women who wrote of natural childbirth experiences were engaged with the process of childbirth as well as with the physiological functioning of their bodies. Dick-Read insisted, indeed demanded, that women become educated about their bodies and about childbirth. When the women became educated, they could control the process and their bodies, something argued by Martin as lacking in women from the earlier centuries. Therefore, by choosing to have a baby by Dick-Read's methods, women were choosing involvement and rejecting alienation.

Conclusion

Dick-Read's theories of natural childbirth changed the boundaries within which women operated. At this time, what was considered by the medical community as normal during childbirth was for women to be drugged and often unconscious. Dick-Read demanded consciousness during labor and therefore offered women a presence in an arena in which physicians were accustomed to having total control (because of the unconsciousness of women). In one respect, Dick-Read demanded women live up to his expectations for them as women—while giving birth—and then live down to his expectations and limitations for them as mothers in the private sphere.

By romanticizing the virtues of natural childbirth Dick-Read contributed to the post-war rhetoric of society's expectations for women—

motherhood. The consequence of his work was that in the post-war period women were pressured by Dick-Read not to take anaesthesia and/or analgesia, while at the same time encouraged to deliver consciously. Where was the option that allowed women a choice and the sense of accomplishment for successfully delivering their children and coming through the delivery healthy themselves? Dick-Read believed he was the only one to offer women this guarantee. In fact he contributed to the pressure that women already felt. A consequence of the writings and teachings of Dick-Read was an added layer of pressure for women to be perfect mothers by delivering their infants painfree, joyfully, and consciously. This he defined and called normal.

Dick-Read believed that eliminating "horror stories" passed on by their own mothers was an important step in educating women about childbirth. In other words, the experiences of women who had given birth and endured pain were viewed by him as a source of other women's pain. Dick-Read believed he had a mission and an obligation to eradicate the fallacies of childbirth. However, in his writings, he sought to overturn centuries of experience, and expected readers to accept his method without question, because he considered what he provided to be the truth. It was Dick-Read's mission to put forward a message that would not only educate women but also engage them in the childbirth process.

At first glance the emphasis on knowledge-on-demand appears to be Dick-Read's contribution to empowering women. Specifically, by providing knowledge there is the appearance that he gave women the opportunity of choice on whether to deliver their babies anaesthetized and unconscious or, as he wrote, calmly, without pain, and in a conscious state. Under closer scrutiny, however, it is apparent that Dick-Read was not empowering women, but instead, persuading them that his method was the only way that was normal for both the mother and the child. When stating that one method was predicated on normality, the unspoken assumption was that if a woman could not achieve this method there was something wrong with her. The pressure to achieve normality was a bitter price to pay for the apparent gift of choosing natural childbirth over childbirth with anaesthesia. In understanding women's roles and the expectations placed upon them, Ann Oakley writes that success in childbirth was measured differently by the medical attendant and the woman delivering the child. Oakley states that women's expectations of childbirth were very important in their overall experience of childbirth:

> For mothers, successful childbirth is often contingent on certain ideas being realized about how birth should be accomplished. If obstetricians

block the realization of these ideas, they may prevent maternal feelings of success and make more likely a pervasive sense of personal failure in the act that is culturally held out to be the primary achievement and proof of womanhood.[20]

Consequently, when Dick-Read put forth his work to the world and claimed that civilization destroyed the way God intended for women to have babies and that the practices of modern medical authorities undermined the natural process of childbirth, women were set-up to expect the perfect birth experience by adhering to his regimen of diet, exercise, and relaxation. These feelings of heightened expectations are evident throughout the letters that follow. Women sought the "perfect" childbirth experience. But the poignancy of the letters are the expectations that Dick-Read established in his writings. He promised that for 95–97% of the women a normal, natural childbirth was possible, and, if it did not happen, then they were the small group for whom, frankly, he held no responsibility. Therefore, in the context of what Dick-Read offered women there was clearly no margin for failure.

In the final analysis, the letters reveal that Dick-Read gave women a language in which to move into the public sphere with their private sphere stories. Women who wrote to Dick-Read were attracted to him not only because of his forthrightness, but also by the atmosphere of anonymity created by correspondence. Safety is deeply imbedded in a relationship conducted in writing. Although the authors of the correspondence express some concern for bothering the doctor, the correspondents' risks were minimal. Therefore, they felt more freedom to write long, detailed, and personal accounts of their pregnancies and labors. Through his writings and theories, he validated them as women, albeit as mothers. He offered women knowledge, and he was an eager audience; this inspired and encouraged them to write to him and trust his advice. As a result, when Dick-Reed wrote back to them it authenticated their experiences as women.

Dick-Read delivered his views of the role of women as mothers in families in a post-war political atmosphere poised for change. Yet he wrote and popularized his theories as a means for preserving the traditional family. He perpetuated a long-standing bias for preserving women as homemakers and the rearers of the future generation. In the end, he contributed to the reinstatement of the private sphere role for women in post-war Britain and the United States.

---

[20] Oakley, *Women Confined*, 27.

In conclusion, the letters are a poignant account of what actually happened to the women writing about childbirth. Regardless of what they considered normal, public or private, they considered it a privilege to be able to give birth and then write their stories. What they did not know when they wrote the letters that appear in Part 2 was that by writing their personal accounts of childbirth, they were contributing to a new chapter in the history of childbirth. They have done so with dignity and integrity and much to the benefit of posterity.

We are able to celebrate their successes, empathize with their frustrations, and sympathize with their failures. The correspondence enlightens our understanding of women's attitudes towards medical institutions, individual physicians, and nurses. We are let into their private lives and are able to understand some of what family life was like for British and American women immediately after World War II. Finally, we can see in many of these letters how society's expectations for them affected what women thought of themselves in the first decade of the post-war era.

Writing about their lives as women and mothers helped them attain a semblance of autonomy in a world that did not readily give autonomy to women. Writing allowed women to make sense of themselves and their roles in life. It gave them authority to step beyond the private sphere and into the public sphere. By writing about their lives in the private sphere and sending their stories to Dick-Read, often with permission for him to use them if he ever published a volume of letters, women blurred the boundaries, even if it was only for the span of time of their pregnancy and labor, thus fusing the separate spheres.

Part 2

Correspondence

Scientific Childbirth

"I was told to stay in bed and I longed for someone to stay with me and help me."

Many women faced a state of uncertainty when it came time for them to give birth. The prevailing medical attitude toward childbirth during the post-war period was that the doctor knew best. This often meant that women should be as cooperative as possible, take drugs, and adhere to the instructions of their physicians and birth attendants. Because physicians preferred the use of drugs they also required that women be hospitalized. Consequently, the letters in this section speak to the isolation and loneliness that many women felt in hospitals. Rather than making it easier for women, drugs often made them feel as though they had failed Dick-Read and most of all drugs made them feel alienated, from their bodies, their newborn infants, and their immediate families. Interestingly, this section provides examples of women who experienced childbirth both naturally and scientifically, which enables a first-hand comparison of both procedures. Dick-Read's role in corresponding with women in this section was to validate their stories of hospital births with drugs as abnormal. He used his correspondence as an opportunity to take his colleagues to task for not learning and practicing childbirth the way Nature intended. Dick-Read, by emphasizing the role of Nature in childbirth, was taking it outside the realm of scientific medicine. The interest Dick-Read generated in his theories was largely enjoyed among the popular audience he cultivated.

Correspondence 1

August 17, 1946
Michigan

Dear Dr. Read:
    Carefully and slowly I am reading every word of your book, 'Child-
birth Without Fear.' In about six weeks I am to have my second child,
my first being three years old. I have almost nothing to recall from her
birth except horror and the other emotional disturbances often accom-
panying ignorance which you repeatedly define. I cannot begin to tell
you what a breath of comfort every new chapter brings me, since I
believe I am an apt candidate for your theories.
    Before my first baby was born when I was twenty-five, I longed to
know the facts of which you speak, and begged my husband who is a
Veterinarian, to inform me of what he knew, since I had come through
college with appalling ignorance as to the functions of birth and its re-
lated responsibilities. However, he, in company with all my mother-
friends, and my over-worked harassed doctor believed in the bliss of
ignorance and happily evaded all my queries, for which I cannot completely forgive them ever for.
    You have so accurately described the inmost feelings of prospective
mothers, that I am warmed just to read about a man who feels so kindly
and works so constructively in a field where we need their protection
and seldom get anything like true understanding. Especially, may I remark about your commentaries on *LONELINESS*, to which I can testify is the most soul-starving experience of all. I was left alone for
twenty-four hours of labor in a strange bare room with only the occasional examinations and hurrying away of impersonal interns. I had no
idea why my husband or some floor scrubber or anyone couldn't say a
word once in that long two days. I tried hard to keep quiet and not
cause trouble, but would gladly have died without even seeing the child
whom I wanted very much
    I have been told that my pelvic measurements are small and have a
record of very painful menstruation's, so am prepared to accept the
fact that I may come under the category of women who need some
extra assistance at the time of birth, but even if this second occasion

Contemporary Medical Archives Centre. Wellcome Institute for the History of Medicine,
London. Grantly Dick-Read, Papers. PP/GDR/D.106. (Hereinafter abbreviated as:
GMAC:PP/GDR/ . . .)

results in as much pain as the first, (and I am certainly trying to condition myself into the belief that it won't), it has been a wealth of good fortune to discover the mental ease your book has given me.

For this baby I have selected a 'specialist' in this large city, who seems most efficient, but completely ignores the fact that I am human and have a mind. I have been afraid to ask if he has an opinion on your theory, but resolve to do so, as I am going to take the book with me to the hospital. I would like to know if there is any advice you can give me which will enable me to help myself through this experiment, as I have only the book for guidance, and purchased it at the advice of a friend a month ago. I should like to try anything you say, and am anxious to tell everyone I know about your suggestions, whether or not they prove applicable to me.

If you have time to reply to this letter, I shall greatly appreciate your consideration. I have written it in care of your publishers, as I have no idea where it might reach you.

Yours sincerely,

27th September, 1946

Dear Mrs.,

I am sorry your letter has arrived so late in England—there appears to have been considerable delay since you wrote it. It is possible, therefore, that you may have had your baby before receiving my reply. If, however, this is not the case I can urge you in a few words to remember that there is no reason at all why you should have any discomfort more than you are willing to bear when your second baby is born.

You have read and become acquainted with the phenomenon of labor. The first stage will require patience, courage and self control so that you may allow the works of nature to have full play without being interfered with by anxieties which give rise to resistance. Remember that the end of the first stage is the most trying phase of labor; you may have considerable backache but it is a purely transient phase and if you will be patient and allow the second stage or expulsive contractions to become established, there is nothing to prevent you having your baby in a normal and natural way, and therefore appreciating the extreme pleasure that it gives a woman to have overcome not only her fears, but her temptations to lose self control.

Just before the baby's head passes the outlet you will again be subjected to certain anxieties, but remember that deep breathing will enable you to maintain in a state of relaxation the tissues of the outlet. I urge you finally to good courage, for if you can exhibit the foundation to a motherhood of which your family will indeed be proud and, what is more, you will have realized that giving birth to a child is the most wonderfully satisfying experience in a woman's life.

I wish so sincerely that you may have someone with you who will understand these things so that you may have a companionable hand and mind to hold on to when you feel that you need support.

My best wishes to you,

Yours sincerely,
Grantly Dick Read, M.A., M.D., Cantab.

Correspondence 2

July 20, 1950
Washington, D.C.

Dear Dr. Read,

I know that I have no right to expect an answer from you because of your heavy schedule, but because during the months before the baby was born I felt closer to you than anyone one else and had such confidence in your method of childbirth, and because I need an answer from you to give me peace of mind, I'm writing in the vain hope you can explain things to me, as I would write to a father.

I read your book over and over before Baby G was born, (She's now seven months) and was so sure it was the 'right way.' It helped in that I had not morning sickness, and never felt better in my life, which is as it should be! I was under the care of one of the best obstetricians in Washington, and had confidence in him and liked him very much.

When it came time for the baby to come, I was so excited that I could at last have my baby the 'right way.' My contractions began at about six in the morning, but were so light that I thought it only a stomach-ache, and went back to sleep. At about three p.m. I was admitted to the hospital, with contractions every twelve minutes or so, but very light to me. About six the membranes broke, and after that they got stronger. By seven-thirty (my mother and husband were visiting me, and mother had always been skeptical) I decided maybe I had better go upstairs to the labor room.

I can remember being wheeled into a dark morgue-like room, and after having my 'pains' checked, was left alone. Then I really lost all control, and began to pain badly, rolling back and forth, and finally asked for something, and was given a shot. That is all I remember except being examined by the doctor at ten-thirty or so. The baby was born at 11:30 p.m. I woke up at 1 a.m. to find myself alone with my hands tied down, and my thighs sore. I was given the information on my daughter and sent downstairs later on. The nurse later told me I rolled around like a monkey in the crib, after the baby was born. (That has always worried me.) By eight in the morning I was sitting up combing my hair, waiting for my husband. (I hadn't seen him yet.) Later I saw the baby, but did not hold her, and felt no connection between us. But I felt fine

CMAC:PP/GDR/D.111

and could have walked home I know, but the doctor didn't even let his patients up for four days! I was in perfect health, he said, so I know there were no complications. I was nineteen at the time, so was certainly young enough. Why then did I loose control then in the labor room? I spend hours wishing that I might relive those few hours and feel the satisfaction of seeing my baby born. I get quite depressed about it the more I think about it, and am afraid of repeating my failure. Why did I forget everything you had taught me? I still have complete confidence that it can work, but feel I failed myself miserably. Can you please help me? I would be eternally grateful if you could reassure me in anyway that I didn't completely fail myself and you.

Sincerely,

22 August 1950

Dear Mrs.,

I have just received your letter dated July 20. It made me turn cold. Unhappily from time to time women write a similar story.

You have read my book carefully. Therefore you realize, I am sure, that one of the chief essentials for the care of a woman in labor is that she should not be left alone during certain phases of the first stage. It appears to me that at a phase we know as 'the second emotional menace,' you began to get pain, and a pain of varying degree in the lower back, and sometimes across the front of the uterus, does occur in 50% of women having their first babies. With properly conducted labor it is easily overcome, but it does demand personal attention and understanding guidance for about half an hour or so. I notice that you, demanding to escape from the situation that was both distressing and unexpected, asked for 'something.' Instead of being given, as my patients are, instruction and assistance to overcome these transient symptoms, you were given a shot strong enough not only to destroy your memory but also destroy all the discrimination and discretion that you had left, which might have enabled you to retain control. You must have been heavily drugged, for I read that it was 1-2 hours after the actual birth of your baby before you regained consciousness. Once a woman has been given drugs which destroy her mental faculties anything may happen. As soon as that influence had worn off naturally you felt perfectly well and wished to get up.

I am not prepared to criticize the actions of my colleagues who are not familiar with the fundamental phenomena of labor. It is their business, and so far as their patients are concerned it is, as you say in

America, 'Just too bad.' Compare, with your experience, what would probably have happened had you been in the Maternity Hospital where the majority of my patients have their babies. At the 'first emotional menace,' which is when the cervix of the uterus is about 3/5th dilated, a nurse, fully competent to instruct you in efficient respiration and relaxation, would have been with you. At each contraction she would minimize your discomfort as you learned how to conduct yourself. At the 'second emotional menace,' just before the cervix is fully dilated still having the companionship of an understanding nurse, I should have been sent for, and had there been any necessity for relief of such discomfort as you might have experienced in spite of the control which I am sure you would have been able to retain, an injection of Demerol, sufficient only to give you a sense of peace and relaxation, would have been administered. About 20% of my primiparous women find this a definite help at this time. Shortly after that you would have commenced to bear down, with the same action and using much the same muscles as if you were evacuating the bowel. But you would not have been allowed to bear down until it became irresistible—that is to say, until you could not help doing it. This constitutes the initiation into the second stage, which is almost entirely free from pain when properly conducted, but which demands physical effort that most women describe as a pleasing ability to help after the long hours of patience and self control exhibited during the first stage. Assuming that the presentation of your baby's head was normal and your pelvis adequate in size, you would have no further discomfort until there was pressure upon the pelvic floor. Then again you might have become conscious of a wave of uncertainty which threatened your control, but this phase that we know as the 'third emotional menace,' rapidly passes if you are instructed in the necessary procedures at this time. You then feel little more except the exertion of pushing until the head is about to be born. With the ultimate dilation of the birth canal you would become conscious of a sensation of burning around the rim of the vulva. It is a threatening feeling, and many women have the impression that they are going to burst, but in reality this does not occur, and again the attendant tells you what to do, how to breathe, and when to exert pressure. In this way a slow and unhurried birth is accomplished in between 80% and 90% of cases with very little, if any, laceration at the outlet. And remember, too, that nearly every woman is delivered in a position which enables her to see her child born, to hold its hands whilst it is crying before the body has completely left the birth canal. My patients tell me the sex of their own child, and as soon as the cord is out they take their babies, wrapped in towels, and nurse and croon over their new possession. In this way the uterus expels with the minimum of hemorrhage the afterbirth within 20 minutes. Within 5 minutes of this final event in labor, the Labor Ward having been tidied, the husband is shown in to see his wife, who is usually a smiling happy girl, without shock or pain, lying with her baby in her arms waiting to greet him.

My patients are up within 24 hours, and on the second day commence certain exercises for the pelvic floor, which entirely precludes the risk of prolapse or weakness after birth. On the fourth day they have a bath, and 99% of them are feeding their babies at the breast; the majority of babies regain their birth weight at or before the end of ten days. They learn to bath and to care for their babies; they learn the art of breast feeding and the preservation of a good supply of milk; they return home fit to carry on the normal duties of their homes.

This is the picture, and there are two in my garden at present as I dictate this letter, playing with a number of children who have gathered for a party, who would relate to you verbatim this experience as having been theirs. Forget your first labor, and when your next child is born find an understanding and sympathetic man who will enable you to enjoy this experience without which no home or family unit can be considered complete.

I do not think you have anything to blame yourself for, and I hope, therefore you will not form any wrong impressions of what can, and I prophesy will, be the experience when your next child arrives.

My best wishes to you. It is my sympathy for you that has prompted me to write so fully to an entire stranger.

Yours sincerely,
Grantly Dick Read, M.A., M.D., Cantab.

Correspondence 3

16 September 1953
Surrey

Dear Dr. Dick Read,

Forgive me for bothering you, but to be perfectly honest, I'm badly in need of your assurance that relaxation is the answer to childbirth without pain. Before I go any further I would like to say that I'm not trying to get a free consultation and that I'm not writing purely to be annoying but after reading your book, 'Childbirth Without Fear,' I genuinely need your advice and although I know that it isn't medical etiquette to do this, I can't quite see how else I can get in touch with you.

To begin with I've been married nearly three years, am 24 years of age, and my first baby was born in May 1952. He was a beautiful boy weighing 9 lbs., perfectly normal, and since birth has never caused me any real anxiety. After reading your book though I'm quite certain that the sheer torture I went through whilst having him was both unnecessary and could have easily been avoided. I've never described my labour or delivery before because quite frankly the sooner I forgot it the better, but now that I am six months pregnant with a second baby, the memory of Infant B's birth keeps me awake at night with the awful recollections of what I'll probably go through again. I'd been out on the Saturday afternoon, the baby according to the doctor was already three weeks overdue, but seeing that it was a first baby, nobody seemed unduly worried, and I felt fine, other than being impatient. My husband incidentally is a Naval Officer and was in New Zealand when all this was happening I was living with my mother as we had no home of our own since being married. On the Saturday evening I had no pains whatsoever, but had a slight 'show' so phoned the hospital where my bed was booked, and was in there within the hour. During the whole of my pregnancy, I'd never felt the slightest bit frightened of having my baby, I was as sappy as a sandboy, and I truly felt that this was the greatest adventure that was ever going to happen to me. On my arrival at the hospital, I was met with the words of 'Oh Lord another one—sit down and wait for Sister.' Sister duly came along and I was taken along to a labour ward, prepared with the usual enema and shave, and then, as I was in no pain, other than a dull backache, was finally taken to the ward, given a dose of revolting tasting medicine and told to sleep.

CMAC:PP/GDR/D.42

This I obligingly tried to do, and eventually fell asleep to be awakened at 5 o'clock am, with the babies being brought to the hospital for their first feed. I was still in no pain, but at 7:30 am while sitting in bed, the membranes ruptured with what seemed to be an awful crack in my back and I went rather faint for a moment. Within a minute or so, I realized that I was really in labour, and other than being scolded by a nurse because of the state of the bed, nobody took any notice. Eventually one of the other women took pity on me, went for Sister and I was helped down the stairs to a labour ward. There I was left alone for two hours frightened out of my wits and literally rolling in pain. Suddenly I felt I must start doing something, so I started to bear down, with the result that my tail was split, my cervix torn and the babe's head was through. . . .I'm afraid that I opened my mouth then and yelled until about half the nursing staff arrived, and within a matter of seconds my son pushed his way into the world. I had an awful attack of coughing just after he was born and the placenta seemed to slip away of its own accord with no trouble. I was then informed that I'd need stitches and that doctor was busy at present, but would be along shortly. My babe was born at 12:45 pm[sic] on Sunday morning. The doctor arrived at 5:30 pm that evening in the meantime nobody came near me either to wash me, give me a cup of tea or to say hello. At 5:30 the doctor arrived to stitch me and decided I should be taken to the theater. The theater apparently was in use so he injected me with a form of cocaine which had not its slightest effect, and then proceeded to put in 20 stitches. I know quite truthfully that the birth of my child was nothing compared to the agony of those stitches and my one fear now is not of pain or of having a baby but of being ripped again and of the sewing up that follows. I genuinely cannot relax. I've tried and tried, because I'm quite sure that its right, and that its the only answer, but everytime I think of this second baby coming, I seem to tighten up all over, and I just can't do a thing about it. I've religiously tried to follow your instructions rather like a drowning man clinging to a straw, but owing to having a prolapsed intervertabrael disc when I was 20, I can't manage it very well as I seem to have a continual pain in my back, and at night I wake up in a cold sweat thinking about it all. Unfortunately, my husband is overseas again, and because of this I must have it in the hospital. We've only just bought our own bungalow, and expenses are rather heavy so that we cannot [spend on] a nursing home for me. Admittedly its a different hospital, in a different area, but to me that's not the slightest help. I feel bitterly resentful that I should have gone through what I did.

I don't truthfully know just what I'm writing to you for, because I'm not a patient of yours. It was just that after reading your book it seemed like somebody giving common sense to the world with both hands. I only hope that other mothers to be have enough sense to take it and I envy them with all my heart.

Yours sincerely,

5 November 1953

Dear Mrs.,

Thank you so much for your letter of September 16 which has just reached me in the mail forwarded to the Belgian Congo, where I am at present making a survey of normal labour amongst the primitive tribes of the continent of Africa.

Relaxation is not the complete answer to natural childbirth, but if you will read again 'Childbirth Without Fear' and in particular the chapters on 'The Phenomena of Labour' and the 'Conduct of Labour,' you will appreciate more fully those things which you must expect to happen during the course of your labour. Relaxing with your contractions in the first stage of labour and between them in the second stage is of great assistance to you, but will not help to a very marked degree unless you are aware of the meanings of your various physical symptoms and mental reactions.

I hope you will have someone with you who will be sympathetic with your aims but remember that patience in the first stage, hard work in the second stage and self-control throughout are all absolutely necessary for you if you wish to achieve your ambition.

Please let me know how you get on. . . .

Yours sincerely,
Grantly Dick Read, M.A., M.D., Cantab.

15 June 1954

Dear Dr. Dick Read,

I don't know whether or not you will remember, but last year I wrote to you (my letter was forwarded to Africa where you were at the time) saying that I was terribly apprehensive about my second forthcoming pregnancy, and how I had read your book, 'Childbirth Without Fear,' but didn't think I would ever be able to look at it from the same view point as yourself. You very kindly answered my letter even though you must have been awfully busy, and asked me to let you know how the delivery and birth were faced when it was all over.

I can never thank you enough for the advice your letter and book gave me and I am enclosing an [excerpt] from the 'Nursery World Magazine.' I wrote them a letter and they published it—I only hope it may encourage other young mothers who are afraid as you encouraged and helped me. Thank you with all my heart for helping me to experience the true fulfillment of being a woman and to achieve motherhood in a way I never dreamed was possible.

I have never been so happy in my life as I was during the three hours that I worked and waited for my baby son—and when he was born. Not even the prospect of a stitched tail could dampen my happiness. Instead I simply gave up a silent prayer of thanks to God for letting my little son be perfect in every way, and also for making me a woman so that I could have children. Also I said a very heartfelt thank you to yourself. For showing me how to get my baby as God must have meant all Mothers to.

Fear *is* the root of all the pain in normal childbirth and if you are happy then there's not time to be afraid.

Thank you—there's nothing else I can say—but thank you so much.

Yours very sincerely,

20 July 1954

Dear Mrs.,

Thank you so much for your very sweet letter of June 15. I am sorry it has taken so long to reply but all my letters are a month behind.

It does give me great satisfaction to read all you have said, and to know that this approach to childbirth which it has been my privilege to introduce to so many women, has been of service to you.

I sincerely hope that in your family life you and your husband and your children may continue to appreciate that there is something other than just a physical act in having a child. Many women have told me that it is the nearest thing to complete spiritual revelation that a woman can possibly experience.

My best wishes and thank you for sending me the cutting [of the article].

Yours sincerely,
Grantly Dick Read, M.A., M.D., Cantab.

Correspondence 4

14 February 1955
Sussex

Dear Dr. Read
. . . I am hoping that you will be able to advise me what to do. I will tell you a little of myself so that it will help you to understand my very deep desire to teach relaxation at childbirth. (I will keep it short!)

I am 38 years. Married. My husband being regular navy. One child [a son], 9 years of age.

Twelve years ago I looked forward to my first pregnancy. I looked after myself, attended regular visits to the Dr. My body was well cared for, but my mind was'nt. [sic] No talks of relaxation. But I thought I knew all there was needed for the birth. I was thrilled when labour began. The waters broke some time later, and that terrified me, as I wondered what was happening. Then a long, and to me a terrible labour began. I was put away into a room on my own for hours, a nurse now and again looked in and asked 'How's it going'. The pains got worse, and I got more frightened, and so I got more tense. After a day and night, I asked a nurse would it be much longer, and she said quite cheerfully 'Oh yes, you've a long way to go yet', I was told to relax, but I could'nt [sic] I had no real idea *how* to.

I was left more hours, I was desperately afraid now, and I did not want my baby, it was no longer an exciting thing, but a terrifying experience. I looked at the large bottle of Dettol on the table with all the instruments laid out, and I fought the desire to drink it. By then I could hardly lift my head off the pillow I was so weak, at last the Dr came, and said it would all soon be over now, and I was prepared for an instrument birth.

When I came around I looked into the Dr's face and knew he had saved my life. I turned my head and saw one of the sisters gown splattered with blood. I was taken to the ward and some-one came and washed my face, and in the mirror I looked at myself and I could see blood splattered across my face. Hours after my little daughter was brought to me, and I was terribly shocked, for she had huge dents in the side of her head, her face was blue, and her little mouth was swollen. I felt so ill I did'nt [sic] care whether I had her or not, and when I did, she felt too heavy, and I was glad when they took her away. I cried in the

CMAC:PP/GDR/D.31

night and I recall saying 'Oh God, why did You have to make such a beautiful thing as birth, so terrible'.

When I was allowed out, I was afraid even to cross a very quiet country lane, and I dragged about with no life left in me.

Five months later I went into a nursing home for the correction of a dropped uterus. Whilst I was in there, my little daughter died from Gastroenteritis [sic]. You will be able to well imagine how I felt after suffering so much for her.

Two years later we went in for another baby, and here I sincerely mean this, I thank God I was brought in contact with your teaching of relaxation, I was given your book "Revelation of Childbirth." I practised relaxing. I went into the clinic to have my baby, having gone in two weeks before it was due, as it was thought I may have to have a Caesarean birth. I was given induction and some hours later labour began. At first I was frightened, memories crowded back of the first birth, but I pulled myself together, and started to relax, doing all you said. Much to my own astonishment I did sort of drop off into naps in between pains in the first stage. Some time after I rang the bell and the nurse came and said 'Goodness your baby is nearly here' I was terribly thrilled. In the later stages I did begin to feel a little frightened and took gas and air. Within a short while my son was born and I felt his little hand in mine. I was sitting up 'made up', and writing an article on his birth and how relaxation had helped me, within a few hours, which I have since sold to a woman's magazine in England, and Australia, when I was there, last year. That birth was as I believe all normal births should be, not frightening but interesting.

Last September I had a Hysterectomy done, my uterus never really recovered from the first birth. Now that I am restored to health I want to teach relaxation. I shall not just only be teaching it, I can speak with experience, because I have proved it does help. I want to explain to the young mothers and nervous mothers to be WHAT is happening, WHY it is happening, and not leave them lying for hours holding baby back with fear by 'shutting' their muscles. I want to teach them why the labour is happening, and to join in with interest, and unafraid.

I feel Dr that apart from the actual birth side, it does'nt [sic] just stop there, it has far reaching affects. It took away a lot of first happiness with my baby. I was too ill to enjoy her. My marriage almost went on the rocks through my intense fear of becoming pregnant again, and finally it had the long reaching affect of ending me up in a gynaecology ward.

Having explained all that, you will see I am not some crank with the idea, but that I do sincerely want to help others to gain from my own experience about relaxation.

Now can you advise me how to set about it? I am neither a qualified midwife, or nurse. I can never afford to pay a fee to become a trained Physiotherapist. I have written to the local Medical Officer of Health a Dr _____ and he was interested, and agreed with the teaching, and hopes in time to get the various bodies concerned together. Apparently most mothers to be in _____ attend at their own Drs but I wonder how many Drs these days have the time to teach relaxation and explain in detail? He advised me meanwhile to contact the matron of the local Maternity Home, which I did, she explained they did have a class for exercises and relaxation but that she would forward my letter onto the consultant, but then I heard nothing, and have come to a dead end.

Today I saw the article on the report of your work, and decided to take the chance and write to you to see if you can advise me what to do next, or is it hopeless as I am untrained? But if that is the case it does seem a pity when I have the ability to speak from experience, and that does carry weight to some one listening if you can say 'I *know* from my own experience'.

Is there anyway I can gain experience in teaching a class? Is there any clinic in London, or near here, which would give me some training? I have very little money, and cannot pay fees for training, but I could afford to travel to London once or twice a week. If I could attend some classes. [sic] My husband gets home at weekends, and my son is at school during the day, so I have plenty of time to study.

I shall be most grateful, if you give me any advise, or at the moment it looks as if the whole idea of my desire to help will just fissile out.

Sincerely yours,

21 February 1955

Dear Mrs.,

Thank you very much for your letter dated 14th February.

It was of interest to me in the sense that just after the First World War, I practised in _____ with a Dr _____ who lived in a large house on the corner of _____ Road. I didn't stay very long however because I went from there to London.

Your letter just embodies everything we have been trying to combat and fight against for the last twenty five years, and I want you to let me use it anonymously in a book of letters that may be published some time to illustrate the appalling treatment women are still getting in a so-called civilized country.

That you should have had a hysterectomy done whilst you are still a relatively young woman seems to me possibly the saddest thing of all. It is women who have had this sort of experience who realise how much there is to be done, and they get the urge to do it to help mothers in every possible way.

Unfortunately at present there is no organized centre where this teaching can be given although, having retired from practice, I am still going around the country lecturing wherever I can and writing as often as I can to make this teaching even more popular.

I believe it might be possible for you to get some very good advice from Professor _____ of _____ Hospital, _____ Street, London (Obstetric Department), or if you can go to London, try and make an appointment to see him. He is one of the few professorial types who is really anxious to have this work carried out and he has adopted an attitude which also means he has got the courage to do it in face of a good deal of aggressive animosity from the Royal College of Obstetrics and Gynaecology.

If you try to see what his reactions are, and don't really get much result, write and tell me and I will see if I can't help you in some other way.

I appreciate your having written to me a lot, but I wish it could have been a happier letter for your sake.

My best wishes,

Yours sincerely,
Grantly Dick Read, M.A., M.D., Cantab.

9 March 1955

Dear Dr. Read,

Thank you so very much for your extremely kind letter of Feb. 21st.

I have not replied sooner, as I have been waiting to see what would happen. I have written to Professor _____, as you suggested, and have received a reply from him, which I will enclose for you to see. You may recall that in your letter to me you did say, if I did not get much result I was to write to you again.

It rather looks as if I am up against it judging from Professor _____'s letter, as I am not trained in anyway. I was glad that you found my letter of interest, and you are quite welcomed to make use of it anonymously in the book of letters, that you speak of. The only thing is would you have to say where the nursing home was that I had my daughter? I do not mind, you knowing, but I would not like it to be known publicly, as after Baby G died the Nuns were very kind to me.

I found it of great interest that you once practised in _____, you must find it very satisfying, looking back over the years, and seeing what great work you have done, you have achieved something really worth while in your life.

Once again thank you for the kindness you have shown me in your letter, if you think it at all possible to help me further, I shall be most grateful.

I am,

Sincerely yours,

21 March 1955

Dear Mrs.

Thank you for sending me Professor _____'s letter.

I was rather afraid there might be some difficulties on the grounds he mentions.

I can only suggest that you find someone who is running antenatal classes in _____, this might be done through the Medical Officer of Health. There it would be possible for you to go as an assistant-learner, that is to say to help in the actual running of the classes and at the same time learning yourself.

That has been done in one or two places and quite successfully and I think it is worth a trial.

I do hope you will find something in due course, and that you will let me know how you get on.

My best wishes,

Yours sincerely,
Grantly Dick Read, M.A., M.D., Cantab.

Correspondence 5

2 December 1955
Surrey

Dear Dr. Read,

I have just finished reading your books, 'The Introduction to Motherhood' and 'The Revelation of Childbirth,' and I have found great comfort in knowing that someone understands the fears I experienced during the birth of my first child eight years ago.

I am expecting my second baby in June and those fears keep coming back. Frankly, I am terrified that this time I will lose my self control.

I had a nervous breakdown two years ago which lost me a great deal of confidence in myself. The psychiatrist I now attend as an out-patient recommended your books to me and after reading them I thought that perhaps you would be able to help me as I do feel so desperately afraid. I may add that the psychiatrist thinks it was a wise decision to have another baby. I had intended having this baby at home after my previous experience in hospital. I broached the subject with my family doctor and he consented to undertake my confinement. However, I gained the impression that he did not welcome the case because of my psychiatric difficulties. This causes me great anxiety as I feel I must have someone to whom I can turn with absolute confidence.

Last time I was left a considerable time alone during the first stage of labour and in every way the birth of my child was an absolute contradiction of your teaching. I don't know whether to go into some hospital or have the baby at home.

I apologize for bothering you with my private problems but I felt I had to get in touch with you.

Yours sincerely,

5 December 1955

Dear Mrs.,

I read with considerable sympathy the letter that I received from you this morning.

It does seem a shame that ladies like yourself should be allowed to suffer from the appalling disease which is the fear of childbirth. It is so completely unnecessary under modern circumstances and in the hands of a good doctor there is less to fear than in an ordinary day in London.

Would you be kind enough to write and tell me all about your first labour—what happened, where you were and all those details. It will help me a lot to be able to advise you as to the best thing to do.

I can quite understand your doctor not being very anxious to take the case of a lady who has suffered from these fears, even to the extent of a nervous breakdown two years ago. I do feel however that your psychiatrist is probably correct in saying that you are wise to have another baby. But if you are properly looked after, the experience of your second birth will have more influence in destroying your fears than anything else. I mustn't stand on the toes of your family doctor, but since I am not writing this as a consultant but only as one concerned with the comfort and happiness of mothers, I feel possible he will forgive my comments.

Until I get another letter from you, I am not quite sure which would be the wisest course to take, but there is an excellent hospital at _____, which is quite near you and the treatment of patients there and the many who have followed my childbirth procedures at that hospital is, I think, as good as any in the London area. But, on the other hand, as I say, I must have more information before I can advise you so I shall look forward to hearing from you again.

My best wishes,

Yours sincerely,
Grantly Dick Read, M.A., M.D., Cantab.

8 December 1955

Dear Dr. Read,

I am very grateful to you for answering my letter so promptly and for your sympathy in my fears. My husband and I thank you very much.

I want to tell you that the breakdown I had was not very severe and that my experiences in childbirth were not the cause of the break although they must have contributed to it.

I had my baby when I was 23 years of age at the _____ Hospital. I had a wonderful pregnancy and I felt extremely fit. I was a private patient sharing the ward with one other patient. I attended our private doctor for antenatal care and he actually delivered the baby. I had no antenatal exercises or relaxation exercises although I had read your book and went into the hospital with quite a happy attitude of mind.

The baby was one week over the expected time and I was admitted to the hospital before any real contractions started. I was admitted at 1 o'clock and put to bed and given caster oil. About 4:30 p.m. the contractions (I will call them pains) began and increased steadily until 7 o'clock. I was then left alone for about 1/2 hour. I was really terrified at this time. A nurse then came and shaved me and gave me an enema and I was again left for a long time. It seemed like an hour to me but I do remember the colic pains and contractions and I was so tense I kept banging my head against the tiles of the toilet wall to help me to bear the pain. The sister returned to my room this time and gave me something to drink which made me sick. However, I was put to bed once more and told to ring but only if necessary.

I wandered up and down the room tense and anxious even praying to die so as to escape my fears. In the end I opened the door of my room which was next to the front door and I remember wishing I dared to go home to my husband for some assistance. However, along came sister and she was extremely annoyed. I was told to stay in bed and I longed for someone to stay with me and help me. By 10 o'clock at night I went along to the labour ward and started the second stage for which I was given gas and air. This part seems rather hazy but I do remember being told not to make a noise like a cow—which upset me because any noise I made was quite involuntary. Then I grabbed hold of sister's hand and she shook my hand away. At that, I felt I must have been a dreadful person to warrant such heartlessness and yet I had made no fuss or noise in front of any one—only when I was in the side room alone did I show any anxiety. However, my doctor arrived and I was given. . . whiffs of chloroform so that I don't remember much. The baby arrived at 1 a.m. I had only one stitch. I know nothing of my baby's arrival and afterwards. I was washed and left in the labour ward until 6 o'clock in the morning all alone so as I wouldn't disturb the other patient in my own ward. I remember telling the nurse that I never expected to come back alive.

The fears and emotional disturbances I felt were horrible and I feel the whole thing was just muddled through and rather sordid.

As far as I know I had a straight forward labour and not too long drawn out but it could have been quite easy had I had someone like you to help me. I have courage and hope that will see me through this time.

I feel I would like to have my baby at home to ensure the support of my husband and perhaps that would help but the thought of being on my own petrifies me. Do you still do confinements? I should be so happy under your care because from all your writings I know you could give me confidence.

Well, I hope I have given you a clear picture of my first labor, and will anxiously await your advice.

Yours sincerely,

P.S. I omitted to mention that we have just moved. . .and consequently have a new family doctor.

13 December 1955

Dear Mrs.,

Thank you for your letter of the 8th December. I am sorry I have not answered it before but I have not been home.

I read what you wrote with a recurrence of all the horror and anger that I have been subjected to for the last thirty years. The gross inhumanity and failure to understand the mind, or indeed the body, of a woman in labor is something which is, to my mind, near to criminal behavior.

I cannot understand why these people who are supposed to look after women in childbirth don't take the care of them which is likely to give a woman a happy birth, a healthy baby and be a healthy woman afterwards. Anyone with the tragedy of desertion, anger, cruelty and misunderstanding to which you were subjected according to your letter, does not deserve to have the privilege of trying to help women to become good mothers.

I notice you are living in _____. Now, if you are there, I think you will find, if you are patient for a bit, there are doctors there who are very keen indeed on carrying out my methods. I am going to look them up in the book, and in a day or two I will get my secretary to send you a note saying who the doctors are whom we know there, and where you can get a midwife who is properly trained and understanding in looking after women in labor.

In the meantime, I do want you to try and practice your breathing and relaxation, and do also get a hold of a little book of mine that is coming out this week, called 'Antenatal Illustrated.' It is 3/6d and will teach you so much, having had a baby badly, how you can improve on it next time. If you would rather have your baby in the hospital there is a good place quite near you where they have delivered several of my patients with complete satisfaction both for the care and management of the woman and her baby and the obstetric side. You let me know what you want to do and when you are picking a doctor to look after you ask him quite frankly and plainly, is he willing to, or does he use the natural childbirth methods, because you want them. If he doesn't that is just too bad. Be firm about it, it is your baby and it is you that is being treated, and there is no reason at all why you should cowtow to treatment you don't want. As a lady wrote to me in a letter this morning, 'I see no reason why we should be bludgeoned into accepting something that is no part of natural childbirth.' It was a very sensible sentence and I want you to know it, so keep in touch with me because if I can be any help to you I should be delighted to do so.

My best wishes,

Yours sincerely,
Grantly Dick Read, M.A., M.D., Cantab.

Correspondence 6

17 January 1956
Middlesex

Dear Sir,

Apropos the recent statement of the Pope on painless childbirth there is a great deal of publicity given to the subject at the moment. I beg you to use your influence to campaign against the out-dated views held by the Royal College of Physicians, and go get your methods accepted as general technique in hospitals, etc.

I write the following carefully and advisedly. Your methods were unknown to me when I returned from abroad to have twins in 1951, but I was confident in the amenities of the large _____ _____ Hospital. Although I am slightly built I gave birth to twins of 8 lbs each, both breeches. I was exhausted and shocked (in every sense) by the first so was unable to expel the second, who was a white asphyxia.

The details I am still trying to forget. I would stress that three years previously I had given birth to an 8 lb girl, at home, with a midwife. I had then no form of anesthetic, was torn, and I suppose had an average painful labour; so I was ready for an appreciable amount of pain, but not the frightful torture of the twins birth. (The gas and air given at this time was so ineffective as to be useless).

If only I had heard of you earlier. . . .If only your methods were generally adopted by hospitals. . . .

I would only add that the mental and physical shock I suffered then has affected my whole life. I have, from his birth, had such loathing for the second twin that the effort to treat him as the others has been a constant struggle. I still, four years later, start from sleep, sweating after a dream that I am again waiting for the twins in that labour ward.

I had already had one child in rough and ready circumstances, I am accustomed to hospital life, I did not expect to be pampered, but I just cannot find any excuse for the inhumanity and downright cruelty that attended my second confinement.

I am writing this in ignorance of your role, in the event of your being a perfectly private practitioner, I will accomplish nothing but, perhaps, to spur you on to greater endeavor on behalf of your pregnant patients, even then, it will not have been wasted entirely.

If there is, at any time, any form of campaign for your methods, my

CMAC:PP/GDR/D.43

time, typewriter, and care are at your disposal. I am not a crank, but sincerely appalled at the thought that other women could so needlessly experience what I experienced, the circumstances that could change a normal, healthy woman eagerly anticipating another baby, into an embittered neurotic, beaten down in mind and body.

I have tried to write this conservatively, with no 'dramatics' and I finish with one incident, that actual snatch of conversation (when I had already started labour) which I think, is typical of the attitude I encountered.

. . . having handed to the authorities the x-ray, which told me I was to have twins, and which had been taken privately by a friend. . .a night nurse pops her head in the door, to see the new patient. . . .

. . .so you're the new one. . .hear you've been having yourself x-rayed. . . .you know what happens to people who have too much radiation. . . .they have abnormal children (and when I tried to remonstrate). . .well I would'nt [sic] like to be in your shoes. . . .

So please continue with your good work, and accept my good wishes for your world wide success, although you appear to have this already, and it is perhaps more a case of a prophet in his country.

Yours sincerely,

24 January 1956

Dear Mrs.,

Thank you so much for your letter of January 17, I am so sorry it hasn't been answered before but my mail, as you may imagine, piles up and piles up and yours has just come to the top.

I am always horrified when I receive letters from women like yourself who tell me this old, old story,—how misunderstanding and ill treatment gives rise to such exhaustion, physical and mental shock, that the attitude towards the child itself is not infrequently altered. This is pooh-poohed by a large number of my colleagues who say 'What nonsense!' and so on.

But then, this is the limitation of their knowledge and that is what we are fighting against.

I have it in mind that probably there will be a great uprising amongst women about this during the next few months and I am going to put your name on the list of those who are willing to help in every way that is possible for them in the circumstances in which they find themselves as mothers of families. It is not only those who have known the misfortunes of childbirth who wish to make this campaign, but those who have known its joys and purposes.

I have had a letter from one lady during this correspondence who has had four beautiful births, all perfectly naturally, simply by reading my book before the first one came, working to [avoid the] doctor who wished to interfere. She was a strong enough personality to be able to push him aside and ask him to watch and not to interfere.

Those are the sort of people who are anxious to give every woman in the country the opportunity of carrying this out and at the same time so turning over the minds of these very conservative teaching schools of obstetrics in this country so that they may work for the well being of women and not just for the pomp and pride of upholding their own rather stale opinions.

So your name goes down, and if you hear from me at any time, know that your letter has not been wasted and I indeed appreciate your very good wishes.

Yours sincerely,
Grantly Dick Read, M.A., M.D., Cantab.

Correspondence 7

20 January 1956
Surrey

Dear Dr. Read,

After reading of the Pope's approval of your method of childbirth I immediately purchased: 'Introduction to Childbirth' and 'Childbirth Without Fear,' and am now saying *if only* I had bought them before I had my little boy. You see I went to clinic, learnt to relax and had my baby *as well* as I could but there were differences which makes me wonder if they do your methods in hospital or merely take those bits which save themselves trouble.

You see I had no idea that the end of the first stage would bring severe contractions. During the afternoon I had been able to sleep and was in no discomfort. About 3 am, I awoke and was horribly sick. A nurse found me and I was taken to the labour ward and left. Shortly after this (it must have been when the membranes went) I suddenly became alarmed at being on my own. I was afraid to ring, I felt I *must* use a bedpan and felt like crying. I held on for as long as possible until I was really distressed and I rang the bell. Sister sounded really cross at me for asking for a bedpan and both nurses seemed in such a hurry I decided that my six children I'd always wanted had now dwindled to one. Nurse said she could see his head and this cheered me amazingly.

This news and their presence restored me and I thoroughly enjoyed the last stage. I was so sleepy between that the Sister said that the infection had nearly knocked me out but after reading your book I see it can be quite normal. Also I had an irresistible desire to hold my breath before letting out a deep breath which exasperated the midwife. Yet I was truly relaxed and felt I must do it. They were full of praise for my efforts which really gratified me and I can only remember three 'pushes' before I was told to hold it and Infant B was born. I was so thrilled and happy and no longer tired I longed to hold him but as he lay there and I played with his little fingers Sister slapped my hand away whereas I see you do let the mothers hold the baby.

Next time I long to do the whole thing with a 'Read devotee.' For me the whole experience would be enhanced by having my husband present and I know most midwives would be shocked even now. Can part acceptance of your theories do you perhaps more harm than good? If I had not read your books I would have gone on imagining I had my baby exactly as taught by you and yet the three things that I disagreed with I find you, too, are in disagreement.

Finally my leg was so heavy that when Sister asked me raise it (for a stitch to be put in) I couldn't and I became known as the mother who draped her leg around Sister's neck.

I was so pleased to see how one man could devote himself to motherhood and am glad that twenty years have brought much of your work to fruition.

Yours very faithfully,

_____ _____, aged 25

P.S. Need I add that my little baby was never any trouble, that I breast fed him happily and even now at 16 months he seems more physically and mentally advanced than those of my friends with their difficult times and bottles! But not any better than those who also believe in natural birth so its not wishful thinking or a Mother's pride.

30 January 1956

Dear Mrs.,

It is nice of you to have written to me so fully, and you know it is the records of ladies like yourself which have meant so much in this teaching. I learn from them and although now we have literally thousands by deducing the important points they raise and the things which require most attention etc. a good deal of the technique of the childbirth program has been evolved.

But don't you think on the whole, it is rather tragic that the nursing profession and of course many doctors have not been taught this thing or even had any experience of it. We have simply got to go on trying in our time because every woman who has seriously approached childbirth in this way and had her baby with the assistance of someone who understands not only what she wants but what labour requires to help it to be carried out nicely, brings such a fund of enthusiasm that it is a great pity we can't disseminate it more fully.

I do like the postscript of your letter. It is so true and I am constantly getting this remark, but unfortunately scientists say there are not controls and you can't see how the child would behave under other circumstances. It is such nonsense isn't it, but that is the sort of thing we are up against.

My best wishes to you, congratulations to your husband, and it sounds to me as though you might be willing to help if there is any conjoined offensive by women, of which I have rumors, in trying to get this more easily available to a large number of people.

Yours very sincerely,
Grantly Dick Read, M.A., M.D., Cantab.

how important it is that we find someone who truly believes that child-birth is normal—not pathological.

That line—'Oh to be in England'—keeps running through my mind, but I'm afraid coming to you is impossible. But please, Dr. Read, if you *do* have a known 'disciple' over here, will you give us his name?

Yours sincerely,

1st April, 1949

Dear Mrs.,

I see that your letter was written nearly a month ago. It has followed me across the face of the earth.

I cannot place _____ in relation to Chicago. I think you would find a sympathetic Dr. _____ _____ of Chicago. He has attended a certain number of patients for me but I am not sure to what extent he has been able to break down the Chicago tradition. I think your wisest plan would be to write to the Maternity Center Association of New York, 654 Madison Avenue, addressing your letter to Miss Hazel Corbin, General Director. She has a great knowledge of all these matters and will, I am sure, advise you to the best of her ability.

My best wishes and I hope you will be successful in your quest.

Yours sincerely,
Grantly Dick Read, M.A., M.D., Cantab.

December 5, 1949
Illinois

Dear Dr. Read,

I am much ashamed that gratitude should be so slow in being ex-pressed. After receiving your kind letter referring me to the Maternity Center Association, I was eventually successful in locating a very good man who believed that the method was the safest and is using it when requested to do so.

The outcome was, as you would expect, perfect. I would not trade the experience for fortunes, and the child, perfect and virile from the moment of birth, has been unbelievably content and healthy. Having had one boy who cried almost unremittingly for the first six months, I was amazed to have the second boy actually seem to enjoy extra-uter-ine existence from birth.

Perhaps the tardiness of this note, recalling a delivery six months ago, will, however, emphasize our continued gratitude to you for your work and its published history.

Sincerely yours,

27th December, 1949

Dear Mrs.,

I may honestly say that I have wondered once or twice how you got on and I am very pleased to hear that your were not disappointed in the arrival of your second boy.

It is such letters as yours that appear to justify ones efforts to impress a simple yet commonsense truth upon the members of my own profession for it is only through them in the long run that women will be able to accept the precepts of an understanding Nature and thereby to mold the activities of a much less understanding Science.

My best wishes to you all and again my gratitude that you have written to me such a pleasing letter.

Yours sincerely,
Grantly Dick Read, M.A., M.D., Cantab.

Correspondence 9

8 January 1950
Sussex

Dear Dr. Dick Read

I am afraid [I] have been rather a long time writing to tell you about the birth of my little Baby last February. Before I start to tell you the details of my own Baby's birth I want to say how absolutely right you are about the complete absence of pain. During ten and a half hours labour I did not have a single stab of pain, nor a sign of back ache which I have heard so much about. If only all women would have faith in what you say childbirth would be something to anticipate with joy not the fear which seems to be so prevalent. I think it is a crime against nature for a normal healthy woman to have anaesthetic during labour and at the moment when her child arrives it robs her of something beautiful which is her birthright. Now I will tell you about my own experience. I had a perfect painless labour. I was radiantly happy the whole time, but against my will they robbed me of my most longed for moment, but I must tell you from the beginning.

At 11 P.M. on February 3rd the exact day on which you said Baby would arrive I experienced the first sensations, I can't describe my feelings at that moment—something which I had prayed for was really coming. For the past week I had walked by the Maternity Home every day longing for my time to come. The moment when I knew my baby was coming was the happiest the most exhilarating [sic] I shall ever experience.

The contractions were very gentle and I was quite comfortable. I arrived at the Nursing Home about 1 A.M. and after what I suppose is the usual routine the Nurse put out the light and left me. The contractions were not very strong and coming almost without intermission but there was no pain.

I would describe the sensations as a sort of pulsing vibration right through the body, something almost volcanic. I had a strange feeling that I was at one with all the vital forces of the universe that I was very near the secret of the human life force.

It was beautiful to be alone. Again how right you are about peace being the great essential. I think a woman could conduct her own labour much better without all the fuss and bother made by those who don't understand her true feelings. I did my best to relax as you had taught

CMAC:PP/GDR/D.38

me and the time passed very quickly. I had an instinct that Baby was really coming so I rang for the Nurse, she had a look and said I was ready to produce my baby.

By this time I was a little tired but still no sign of pain.

My feelings on the way to the labour room were very happy because a most longed for moment was drawing very near. In due course the Doctor arrived (if only it had been you) he was very pleased to find me so happy and comfortable. I looked at the clock and noticed it was five A.M. The Doctor talked with me explaining what was happening and I found it very interesting. Then just as you said in your book I began to grow sleepy. I went sound asleep between contractions but became wide awake in time for the next one, a wonderful phenomena.

Then to my utter amazement the doctor suddenly suggested giving me an anesthetic and using forceps. I became wide awake in an instant, I said certainly not I am comfortable happy and without pain why should I have that. He replied that the Baby was too long coming that it had turned the corner but now seemed unable to move further, he feared it would suffocate if left much longer. It was then 7 A.M.

I said, but some people are two days in labour I have only been eight hours. Why do you say it is too long? He replied yes but the women who go two days are in the first stage, the second must not be prolonged.

Absolute panic took possession of me, I pleaded for a little more time then I grew angry and refused to have anything. I awoke to frantic effort but still baby did not move.

For the next two and a half hours I fought against having an anaesthetic, another Doctor and two Nurses came in I resisted all their efforts and refused to sign the paper. Then the Doctor who was really very kind and patient told me the Baby's heart-beats had dropped from 112 to 106, he said if I resisted further it would be born dead.

What was I to do? If you had been present all would have been so easy because I should have taken your word unhesitatingly but as it was I could not be sure that forceps were really necessary, I had no confidence in those around me.

But I was afraid to hold out if my little Angel had been born dead I should never have forgiven myself. So I surrendered and all the heart went out of me. I was only unconscious a short time, just half an hour from nine-thirty until ten A.M. I must have been coming round when they took the Baby away because I had a clear vision of a little screwed up face and a little bundle wrapped in a blue blanket, I also saw the Doctors leave.

When I fully awoke I was being washed. I can't tell you my feelings then when I fully realized that it was over, the moment which could never come again. My little one who should have been welcomed by a flood of love and joy had been brought into the world in darkness and sorrow. I turned my face into the pillow and sobbed.

They thought I was depressed from the anaesthetic but it was not so, at that moment which should have been one of supreme joy to look back on all my life, I was heartbroken. I had hoped and dreamed that when my Baby came I should be able to touch the little head I wanted to feel the little soft thing so loved and waited for, to know the miracle of joy and peace which should have been mine. As it was I did not see my baby for a day and a half and every time I looked at her little head I visualized it gripped by [a] hideous instrument my reaction was stupefication. I used to lay for hours just staring at the wall.

The other thing I most hoped for was to feed my Babe. To see the little thing nestled against my breast and to know she depended on me for her life and well being was a beautiful experience. I shall always remember her like that. But before the end of my twelve days at the Home my milk began to go and when I arrived home it went completely. I tried every-thing I knew of to get it back but it was no use, so again I was cheated.

When I look at my little girl now and remember all the joy she has brought me during the last twelve months it seems wrong to write of sorrow as I have done in this letter, God has given me such a treasure I should never complain of anything again. But I must tell you what hap-pened and how I felt at that time because it again proves you right.

A Natural Birth is a happy beautiful experience free from pain. I am very grateful to you for all you taught me I wish every woman would believe as I do.

Please go on with your wonderful work and one day know you will win the fight and the whole civilized world will believe that you have discovered the truth, the shadow will be lifted from childbirth and it will become what nature intended. My own experience would not have been so bad if someone had understood my feelings but they all seemed to accept anaesthesia as the normal thing and to wonder why I did not want to have it. I am afraid this letter is not very academic but it comes straight from a woman's heart and if any part of it is useful to you please quote it with my full name and address if you wish.

My little girl is a lively Baby healthy, happy and so good I wish [I] could bring her to see you. I think her good health is due to the fact that I followed your instructions as to diet, exercise and relaxation during the waiting period. You used to tell me she would be contented be-cause I wanted her so much.

Wishing you every success in the coming years—

Yours sincerely,

P.S. I forgot to mention something rather important. My Baby's birthweight was five pounds, fourteen ounces. Such a light weight but she was beautifully made although small.

30 January 1951

Dear Mrs.,

I have wondered many times how you got on and was delighted to have your letter. Perhaps no one better than myself can imagine your happiness.

The description that you have sent me of your thoughts and feelings tallied very closely with what I believe to be the normal emotional response of a woman who has a natural outlook upon the birth of her child. I can only wish you all happiness. I have already told you how much I admire the courage of your undertaking.

Yours sincerely,
Grantly Dick Read, M.A., M.D., Cantab.

Correspondence 10

August 5, 1953
Whereabouts not indicated—somewhere in Southern United States

Dear Dr. Read

This letter was begun on June 22nd, the birthday of my first child, Baby G, who was born about four o'clock that afternoon. That night, being far too much excited and having so very much to think about, I could not sleep. It occurred to me that I would like very much to write to you, and so I began my letter. . . a letter of *thanks*. I had read *Childbirth Without Fear* and the seeming rightness of what you had to say, and beautiful way in which you said it struck home with me, and I determined then to have a 'Read Baby' if I could! I thank you with all my heart for the most incomparably wonderful experience of my life. It was *you* who made it so! *Thank you* for writing that book!

Well, my daughter has kept me pretty well occupied during these past six weeks, and so our letter has been delayed, though I've been writing parts of it ever since it was first started! I should like now to tell you of my experience for I hope, and feel, that you may be interested to hear.

I didn't go all the way without anesthetic, I'm sorry to say, for now I know it was completely unnecessary. But to start at the beginning: I had asked my doctor whether or not he ever prepared his patients for natural childbirth, but he said that he didn't. . .didn't have time. He said I could get your book and read it, (which I already had!), and that he would not stand in the way of my efforts when the time came. I satisfied myself with this. (He, and all the other doctors in this vicinity are exceedingly busy due to the fact that we live in what was once a sleepy southern area but which now is seething with 'H-Bomb' Plant workers. The site for the plant was ordained by the U.S. Government, and thus an influx has occurred of many thousands of people. . .plant-workers, wives, families, and all their various and sundry ailments! My husband, _____, and I are, in fact, a part of the herd!)

The pregnancy was flawless. I was never sick a day, and on the contrary, had never before enjoyed such health and spirits! I would wonder at myself for being so happy! I felt a love for all human-kind it seemed, and was so *proud* to be pregnant!

My first-stage labor began (two weeks early!) at about 2 o'clock A.M. on the day Baby G was born. I felt the small cramp-like feeling, then, at

CMAC:PP/GDR/D.107

about four-minute intervals (on the average) for approximately the next
thirteen hours. During the last hour the feeling became gradually more
severe, but 'perfectly bearable' as you say. I felt it all in the lower portion of my *back*, and tried pressing it there as I remembered you had
written about that, in the case of one woman who had felt discomfort
in her back. This helped. It was rather funny because all morning, (I
went to the hospital at 7 A.M.), I was strolling around the halls, periodically pressing my back as I chatted with the nurses or my doctor,
who happened by every now and then during the stroll! My husband
had brought me to the hospital that morning but we decided he should
go home for a while, and to bed, as he had just come home from work
when I began feeling the contractions (he works on a shift-schedule,
and that week was on the 4 p.m. to Midnight shift) and thus had no
sleep. He came back to the hospital, then, about noon and, (except for
the delivery-room), was with me all the rest of the time. I was so happy
they allowed this!

The doctor came to see me in my room just before noon. I must
have acted quite impatient about the waiting, for he asked me if I wanted
him to 'hurry me up'. 'No', I said, and then asked him what he had
meant exactly. He said he meant he would break my water. I didn't see
any reason for that and said so, and so he left.

I lay in my bed all afternoon next to [my husband] who said he always knew when a contraction was going on by the way I would seem
to sink into the bed, hands go limp, and face suddenly 'sag from my
cheekbones'! At first, I pretended that you were sitting by my bed too.
. . telling me what to do. (My doctor was busy all the while in the delivery-room and elsewhere, for he delivered, I think, four or five babies
counting mine during the time! He came in, of course, from time to
time, to see how I was progressing.) Then, I'm afraid it became harder
and harder to summon up your image, and so to keep my mind occupied I began to concentrate on the birds singing outside my window!
(Such warbles and trills! I'll never forget them!) My doctor is really very
kindly, but he loves to tease. (I don't wish to paint a bad picture of him.
I do believe him to be an excellent medical doctor, and I like him!) We
had been bantering back and forth that morning about 'the Read
Method', and I had told him how disappointed I was that he was not a
practical believer in it. I suppose I was rather flippant really. Anyway,
just when I began to feel it had been a very long day, and that I was
quite tired of waiting to 'help', he came in to see me. He asked how I
felt, and I replied, 'fine'. He said, 'You don't seem so sure of yourself as
you were this morning'. If, at that moment I had happened to have a
double-barrel shot-gun handy, he would have 'gotten it', for that re-

mark, *both barrels*!! However, I knew he didn't understand, and so I told him I was just going to have to see what would happen. I knew, too, that was his way of feeling me out, so to speak, to see whether or not I really wanted to go on with it. . .for he, I think, really believes that to allow a natural childbirth would be inhumane!

I happen to be RH Negative, (my husband is Positive), and as soon as the doctor left a young girl came flitting in. . .the technician [sic] who had taken my blood for a Coombs Test a month previous. She had told me then that she *too* was RH Negative, and how worried she was about it, and wasn't I worried too etc., etc.! Well, all this was repeated and enlarged upon as I lay in my bed trying to think of anything but my RH Factor! I could see my husband's jaw tensing as he listened to my friend's chatter and its lucky for her she left when she did! She didn't really bother me because I knew she didn't know what she was doing.

Well, that happened about 3:20, I should say, and pretty soon after that, and for about the next fifteen minutes or so, I was what I call 'exceedingly uncomfortable'. I don't use the word 'pain', because it wasn't like having a tooth drilled which to me is painful! I had begun to lose control of myself and to think I'd be all night at it. I didn't know whether matters would get worse, or just *what*. (It was the 'pain period', but I didn't think of that.) (I wish I had!) [My husband] was still with me and trying to help me, but 'you' were gone, and even the birds seemed to have vanished! I couldn't seem to make myself relax very well, and tears came into my eyes. I told [my husband] I'd had enough and please to tell them to bring me something now. [My husband] balked for a while! He asked me if I wanted to hold on to him, and I tried, but I couldn't seem to grasp his hand. He patted mine, and said, 'Now Honey!. . .Now Honey!' Finally I felt I'd had absolutely enough and insisted that I wanted something. . . I was very tired of it by then. . .'an aspirin, anything!', I said. My husband is a clever soul. He went out into the hall and returned shortly, *not* with the anesthetist, but with. . .*an aspirin*! (As you see, he is as much interested in natural childbirth as I am! Also, he knew how much I wanted to have the baby that way, and judged the aspirin a pretty good compromise, or temporary measure at least!) It was pink and I thought it must be bogus and said so. 'However', I said, 'Maybe it will do some good psychologically', and when I had time downed it voraciously.

Just at that time my water broke. I was so relieved that it finally had! Some of the nurses were there, (they were all kind and very much interested). Suddenly, there was tension among them and one of them cried out, '*Get the stretcher!*' She had seen the head! O glorious relief, I thought, at last I can help! Such a flurry! Onto the stretcher, good-by to [my husband], (and two neighbors who had got in somehow!), down the hall, and into the delivery-room! My doctor was already there. *Nothing happened!* The head had withdrawn itself, and the doctor hardly believed it had been seen at all. It certainly wasn't visible then! While they deliberated about what to do with me, I subsided into a state of resignation and waited almost happily in that cool place. It was air-conditioned and blissful after the heat of my room and the heat of our late excitement! I said something about it and one of the nurses asked the doctor if I couldn't be left there. He said not, and back I was trundled to my dear old bed! [My husband] was not there, but they got him back again and everyone else left. I had two more severely uncomfortable dilation's and determined I *must* push! I didn't know whether I was hindering or helping, but I *had* to do something. I had lain there idle long enough! So, for these last two 1st-stage contractions, (as I think they must have been), I pushed with all my might. It didn't *seem* to hasten things at all, but was such a relief somehow. Then [my husband] saw me crowning. He dashed out into the hall and grabbed a nurse, (we knew her, as it happened, for her husband works at the plant too), and the two of them came flying back. '*GET THE STRETCHER*' again! The nurse ran to tell the doctor, who was helping to get another girl on to *another stretcher* bound for the delivery room! He could not believe I was ready, for he had just examined me a few minutes before. However, as the other girl was unconscious and not in any hurry he came to look at me, still unbelieving. Another contraction. . . as I figure, the first in the 2nd-stage. 'Push!, they told me, and I was not slow to obey! I heard one of the nurses say to my doctor, 'Now isn't this better than having them kicking and hollering and out of their heads?' He didn't answer her. I was a bit fretful, however, in all the uproar, and testily told the doctor I wished he'd *please 'quit poking me'*! He saw my Baby G's head then, and up onto the stretcher I was heaved for the second time.

I was feeling completely different by now. They rolled me out of the room, and I started to draw up my knees. A hand from somewhere knocked them down again. (There seemed to be hundreds of people in white all around!) 'Can't I raise my knees,' I asked?

'Not out here, Honey'. (Everyone calls everyone else 'Honey' in this part of the world!)

'I've *got* to!', I said, and with that 'bore down' with the second tremendous 2nd-stage contraction. Every fiber seemed to be straining. It was not painful, only immense. I was awe-struck by it. I wondered at myself as I heard the noise I was making. . .something between a grunt, a groan, and a roar. . .very loud and completely beyond my control. (Up until then I had at least kept quiet!) That subsided, and I looked around for my husband, (we were still in the hall), for I wanted to wave good-bye again. I only saw some strangers way down the way looking startled! 'Where's my family?', I asked, for by this time I was including the neighbors as family too! Neither [my husband's] nor my parents are living now.)

'They're gone' the doctor said.

'Oh'. I lapsed into that dormant state of which you speak, and remember thinking how my doctor seemed devoid of insight!

I must have been nearly exhausted, though I didn't feel tired, only remote and heavy. A voice in my ear said very kindly, 'do you want to keep on being brave or do you want to take a little something now?' It was my doctor's voice. He was holding me beneath the shoulders, helping to lift me off the stretcher. Ah, the delivery-room again, I thought abstractedly. My head flopped forward and I thought to evade his question. At this point, I wanted to 'take a little something' quite heartily, (or so I thought), even though I knew I wasn't in pain. I seemed to have lost my reason somehow, for I had forgotten that the moment for which I had waited for nine months was now at hand. . . that this was the time to be awake and aware, the time to greet my baby, to be with those who would see and hear her for the very first time. My doctor's question was still revolving in my mind and I sought for what I wanted to answer. The way in which it had been phrased irked me. . .about 'being brave'. . . entirely the wrong conception of the situation at hand! (I had no fear at any time.) Finally, I answered only, 'I want to see my baby.'

The voice, kind and quietly persuasive said again, 'Well, but let's take a little something now; I think it's time we did.'

I looked at him and saw concern and pity in his face. . . as if he wanted more than anything to 'put me out of my misery!' I gave in.

'I don't want to be put way, way under!', I said. I kept looking into his face, appealing I don't know just for what.

'Well, I can give you something that will only last for about twenty minutes'.

'Twenty minutes?', I asked, weakly considering.

'Twenty or thirty,' he said.

'All right.'

With that the order was given and I was put upon the delivery table. I lay there in that semi-torpor between contractions, absolutely *NOT* in any pain whatever.

The other girl was, by the way, on the delivery-table next to me. She was also ready to deliver at any moment, and by the same doctor. She had been doped all day long, as I could hear from my room, and thus was much slower than I in the second stage.

We were having equal attentions, there in the delivery-room, until suddenly, it was all 'Mrs. _____! Mrs. _____! Mrs._____! As they were furiously strapping my legs and arms, dumping Methiolate, (or some such substance) over me, and doing I know not what besides, I said once more, 'I don't need anything now!'

My doctor replied, 'Not Now. . . .' and left the sentence hanging.

Another tremendous contraction occurred at that moment, the third and last I felt. There were only four all together. Just at this time the shot must have been given. I remember saying, 'God damn!', and knew I hadn't wanted to say it. I heard the nurse above my head say, 'Oh she said. . . . !'; I felt the knife out, and the head be born. That is all I remember, and neither the cut nor the birth of the head was painful. Just as the head was coming through I had a sort of vision. . .like swimming up from the bottom of a lake, and just before breaking the surface, seeing the sun's rays shining down through the water. I experienced that 'bursting' feeling of which you speak, but I recognized it immediately from your description, and it did not alarm me.

I awoke only about *five* minutes later, just in time to see the *after-birth* being delivered! I sprang up on my elbows and asked eagerly, 'Is that the baby?!', for I'm sure, had I been told it *was*, I'd have thought it *beautiful*!

The doctor, however, said hastily, "No, no, this is the after-birth. . . the baby has already been taken to the nursery.'

'Oh', I said, sinking back disappointed into my anesthesia.

I was in the delivery-room a total of ten minutes only, and for *two* of these minutes, as my doctor later told me, I was in the 2nd-stage labor under anesthetic. Wasn't it a ridiculous pity? Though the time while conscious was so short, I do not mean to imply that I was 'put under' without my own consent I could at any time during the period, brief though it was, have absolutely refused to take the shot, and my wish would have been granted. The nurses were all 'for me', (or for *you*, I should say!), and my doctor had promised me he would not force anything on me and I'm confident he would not. However, though I missed my 'reward', that of seeing my little daughter and holding her while she was yet a part of me, I do not think she had time to be doped, or perhaps only a very little, and that after all is the real blessing. She is so precious to us! Very bright seeming, and active. (She turned over at the age of one week, and has been doing that, and 'creeping' all over her crib ever since!) She was quite tiny, having weighed 5 lbs., 7 3/4 oz. when born. I feel sure it was unnecessary that I should have been cut for such a tiny infant's passage into the world. Of course, I have no knowledge on this subject, and oughtn't to pass judgment on what happened. Perhaps my doctor is one who believes it is right to cut in every case. I have only two stitches, however.

You are probably wondering about the girl on the other table! I was told later that she did not deliver for another two hours.

I was brought back to my room, where my husband and a nurse, (our friend), were waiting. The doctor came in shortly too. I do not remember talking to them, though my husband says I carried on a rational enough conversation. I *do* remember that our child was brought in and lain upon the bed beside me. She was looking right up at me with her sweet little puffy eyes, then scarcely open! I rose up on my elbows over her in a paroxysm of delight and wonder!

'*OH HONEY*!!', I cried, flinging my arms around my husband's neck and kissing him!

They swiftly removed the baby after this outburst, as I watched in sorrow, and shortly thereafter I sank into sleep. All over. All beginning!

The experience was fascinating and I think of it with real joy even though I fell down on the job at the last. I read your words, and I believed them. But now I *know myself* from *experience* that childbirth can not only be perfectly 'bearable', but can and by all means *should* be *enjoyed*! I enjoyed it, really, all of it, except perhaps that bad fifteen minutes at the end of the first stage when, I feel sure, had someone been able to say, 'Good! Now the first stage is almost over! Soon you will be able to help bring your baby into the world!', I would have handled it quite differently, and have been able to enjoy that part with all the rest. And in the delivery-room, if I could only have known the baby was coming so soon! I will enjoy it all *next* time! For you see, experience was my teacher, and has already prepared me for my next baby's birth! I want six more, and they shall be 'Read Babies'!

One more incident: The next day, my very first visitor was my RH Negative acquaintance of the laboratory! 'I just *had* to see that RH Negative baby!', she said! 'I looked at her before I even went to work!'

'And you see', I said, 'she is perfectly all right!' I tried to make her understand there was nothing to worry about. . .that *I* wasn't worried. If it should happen that either she *or* I ever had trouble with our RH Factors, why, after everything else had been tried we could certainly adopt our children! She seemed half-way satisfied with this, and after an 'Oh Kid, I hear you did just grand!', flitted out of the room.

The doctor then entered and we talked about it a little, but he is rather uncommunicative, and was then. I know he was interested. (I'm determined to 'convert' him!) If he was interested, he would never have admitted it though. He said gruffly, 'I think anybody's crazy to want to have a baby without anything!' I started to say, 'Well you don't know what you're talking about. . .you've never had one!', but I restrained myself! He has taken excellent care of us, I know that.

Ever since, I've been happily spreading the word to my friends. . . your word. There must be many hundreds of women who thank you for your life's work, and I like to think of the many millions who will from this time forth. I hope you think of that too sometimes, for it is right that you should realize the inestimable worth of what you have done, and that women everywhere know and give you their real thanks.

Sincerely,

P.S. I wrote to the editors of TIME magazine for your address, and they not only sent it, but their congratulations on the birth of our baby!

2nd February, 1954

Dear Mrs.,

Thank you so much for your letter of the 5th August which followed me all over Africa before reaching me, for I have been touring Central Africa carrying out a survey of the habits and customs of childbirth amongst the 'unwesternised' peoples of that continent.

Your letter gave me a great deal of pleasure to read although everything did not turn out as you desired you quite obviously knew what you wanted and had you received the help and understanding so essential from one's attendants at this time I know you would have experienced in all its aspects the full joy of seeing your baby actually born and holding her in your arms at once, though I must say I was appalled to read that your legs and arms were 'furiously strapped down'. I hope, therefore, when you have another child you will be able to overcome the setbacks of this occasion, or should I say when you have your other five!

You did not put your address on your letter so I am sending this to you c/o Time Magazine, and hope that it will reach you eventually. With it I send to you, your husband and Baby G my very best wishes, and please congratulate your husband for me on his very sensible outlook, which in itself did so much to help you.

Yours sincerely,
Grantly Dick Read, M.A., M.D., Cantab.

Section 3

The Struggle between
Consciousness and Unconsciousness

"I had beaten that needle to the punch! Hallelujah!"—

For women who read Dick-Read's books and prepared on their own for labor, it was a moment of supreme achievement when they delivered their babies naturally. The preparation included adhering to a healthy diet, following a strict regime of exercises, and setting aside periods of time for concentrated relaxation. Women wrote not only of their childbirth experiences but also about the close feelings they had with their babies after a natural childbirth. This group of letters points to the sense of accomplishment that women felt when they achieved all that Dick-Read "promised" them. In many cases, they succeeded in their efforts to accomplish natural childbirth over the objections of their physicians. Interestingly, in some of the letters expressions of gratitude for Dick-Read's work and writings led women to credit him with their success. When writing to women in this section, Dick-Read stressed the importance of the role of the Divine. He wrote that natural childbirth was God's intention, indeed, His gift to all women. Only the 3% who could not achieve natural childbirth were exempt from His watchful eye. In other words the "normal" also equaled the "blessed."

Correspondence 11

September 24, 1948
Michigan

My dear Doctor Read,

My doctor and I agreed in the delivery room that I should write you. What a pity that I had to have my fifth child before I knew how to have them. If I had read 'Childbirth Without Fear' sixteen years ago I would have been spared hours and hours of utter torture because I worked against the contractions. And I would have avoided the deep episiotomy that I had to have with each. My doctor said I was so relaxed I wouldn't need it this time but for the scars that wouldn't give; and this was an 8 lb 15 oz boy. I was his second patient to try your method; the first not being able to follow it because of the position of the baby. Dr. _____ was most cooperative having the anesthetist help me in other ways, and reminding me once or twice of what Dr. Read would say to do now. One of the doctors with whom I have talked since said it would not become a universal method tho' as long as half the women who came to him ask about what anesthetic he would use, the very first question. I have had scopolamine with three and can honestly say I was far better off without it both during labor and in the days that followed. It or the agony even seemed to affect my mentality making me so absent minded for about a month. However, I don't know that I could have stood my two severest times without any anesthesia as it at least relaxed me between pains. I have always labored eleven to twenty-six hours. This time it was six from starting contractions to delivery. My doctor ruptured the membranes an hour before birth, as my contractions had almost ceased. I had a few good hard contractions and I won't say they or the preceding ones were painless—then only four or five second stage which really weren't as painful but good hard work. It was indeed a thrill to see my little son - upside down - and hear him start to live in the world. I expelled the placenta in about five minutes. But then it required three shots of Novocain to deaden the area enough so that stitches didn't hurt terribly. It had to take so many and I felt all but about the last three.

I felt on returning to my room that I must call everyone in to tell them how to have their next baby—and I have told everyone within earshot, and even written two English cousins to be sure to study your method.

CMAC:PP/GDR/D.109

One thing that has helped me to regain my strength quickly is getting up the second day. I didn't have time to lose strength lying in bed. They are doing that in most maternity hospitals now. This has been much too long but as an enthusiastic supporter of the Read method I felt I must express my gratitude and describe my case.

One you may not have heard about—and supposed to be true—tells about a woman reading a book on the delivery table, telling the nurse to hold it a minute so she could take hold of the handles, and deliver, then continuing her reading. Another I heard in the delivery room, the woman delivered then got up and walked back to her room. Both [by the] Read method.

Most gratefully,

4th November, 1948

Dear Mrs.,

It was very charming of you to write to me about the delivery of your child and once again, as so often, I am happy to be able to send a message of good will to your great country. Every week I have letters from somewhere in the United States saying how much they have appreciated the procedures which we in England are rapidly adopting as general. It is not of course that I allow any woman to believe that her labor will be painless but I do tell them that many labors are completely without pain and that all normal labors can be conducted so that any discomfort may be immediately dispelled and that the final stages should be so free from discomfort that she may have the happy sense of achievement that seeing her baby brings to a healthy minded woman

Curiously enough I am today answering other letters from Michigan, and since it appears that your doctor at the _____ _____ Hospital is interested in this method of delivery, if you can obtain his permission to send me his name I would like to communicate with him as from the purely medical point of view there is a good deal of unpublished work which might assist him from the Doctor's standpoint to a fuller understanding of some of those phenomena which have not yet been fully appreciated by ourselves. Again thank you very much for your kindly contribution.

My best wishes to you. I must add that it is nice to hear of a woman having six children. In my last 500 cases there was not a single woman with more than three.

Yours sincerely,
Grantly Dick Read, M.A., M.D., Cantab.

Correspondence 12

28 January 1949
Massachusetts

Dear Dr. Read,

This is to express my heartfelt appreciation to you for taking the time and energy to write Childbirth Without Fear for us helplessly ignorant women who love and want babies naturally but for whom no one but you, has ever bothered to teach or instruct. (I hope that long sentence doesn't wind you.)

Doctor, I am so happy with this last birth that I'll never be able to adequately express my thanks. I first learned of your book through the newspaper column writings of one Dr. William Brady. He is high in his praise of you and writes of you frequently.

I have always wanted a baby without anesthesia but each time the point was reached where from the waist down the pain was excruciating, and I had ether. Then came my day of liberation, the day I read your book! I was thrilled with it and knew that what another woman could do, so could I.

You would have rated me probably as the most uncooperative type of patient. In the first place I could not stick to your meatless diet. My husband insists on meat three times a day. . . . Regarding the exercises, I did them for about a month but they tired me terribly during the day and at night I was too tired to do them. However, on the relaxation I scored a 100%. I relaxed for five and ten minute periods several times a day and before sleeping at night.

This was my third baby in less than three years. She arrived ten days early, which I expected because my other babies were one week and three weeks early. Labor started at ten fifteen on Saturday night with contractions three minutes apart from the start. I telephoned the doctor who lives twenty miles west of Boston (where the hospital is located) and my husband and I started right out since we live thirty miles south of Boston. Of course the roads had to be icy, but it was fun. I put the light on over the car clock so that I was able to time the contractions. I was sitting on the front seat and had on my blessed corset without which I could never get along, and I did my best to relax. The contractions were one and one half minutes apart when we got there and they weren't bad at all. In fact, when we came in the door, the nurse asked us if we'd mind waiting a little while as she had something she wanted to do! My husband told her that would be fine if she were prepared to deliver. I don't think she believed us but she assigned me to a room and my husband sat down to rest. (He is a highly excitable man.)

Twenty minutes after admission, I was in the delivery room and fifteen minutes later I was back in my room, my husband had seen the baby and we were talking together. Doctor Read, it was a miracle, it made me proud to be a woman, I was supremely happy!

I first saw my Doctor as I rolled into the delivery room. He asked me how I was doing and I answered that I'd tell him later, right then I was busy relaxing! I had felt all along that he was a 'doubting Thomas' although he had assured me we would do it exactly as I wanted. During my last visit to him, we were discussing the delivery and he just abut crushed me when he said he would only use Novocain in the perineum so that I wouldn't feel it when he cut me! My heart fell right down to my feet. After all the harping I had done on *no* inducing (good idea he thought because of the distance we live from the hospital), *no* anesthesia, *no* forceps and *no* cutting! My doctor is by the accepted standards hereabouts, one of the best obstetricians. He delivered my other babies with forceps and I have two lovely scars in my perineum. One of them runs up along the anus, the other is about half as long. Remembering the discomfort of the stitches, I didn't want to be cut no how!

In the months before the birth there were many nights I woke and prayed that no one would put a needle into me when I wasn't looking. But to get back to the delivery, the last part of the first stage wasn't bad at all. While I was doing my best to relax, the nurse slipped a long cotton bag-like stocking on my left leg but she never got one on the other leg, I was much to busy by that time pushing little Baby G out. It was at this point I nearly lost my nerve. I squeezed my eyes shut and in doing so remembered 'eyes open' so I opened them. I asked for the ether cone and forgot to relax between the first two pushes. After the second push I remembered about relaxing again and put the cone aside. The third push got the head out and the fourth and last push the rest of the baby. The nurse put her hand on my belly and the after birth was out. Then I sat up and saw my baby and heard that funny sobby cry. I nearly burst with pride! I had wanted a girl in the worst way so that I could name her after my mother-in-law who died recently, and here she was! I tore a little but, small wonder but two stitches repaired me.

This was the first baby's birth that my husband had been able to wait for and he saw her before she had been bathed or put into the nursery and he was jubilant! You don't mention the father at all but I believe natural birth affects him too. [My husband] looks at me and behaves toward me as though I were the most precious person in the whole world. He has always been the only and most wonderful husband for me and now there is an added quality I can't define—but I like it and you are responsible for it and I thank you with all my heart.

Regarding the after affects, there haven't been any. I was up and about five and one half hours after the birth. I left the hospital on the seventh day. Since I got home I have carried on as usual taking care of the three children and a seven room house. There is one thing I think helps a great deal and this is a good, sturdy, boned corset.

That is my story Dr. Read. I have written it so that you might know that even in Boston, three thousand miles away, your book has given knowledge and happiness to one woman and in all probability to many others here also.

When I have my next baby I'm going to enjoy every minute of it. I won't get scared and I'll have more confidence in my doctor (if he'll ever take care of me again) and golly, I can hardly wait!

Sincerely yours,

30 March 1949

Dear Mrs.,

I was very pleased to read that through reading an article in the newspaper you were persuaded to study more deeply my obstetric doctrine. It does give me great pleasure to know that women can have happiness instead of horror in childbirth.

The story of the birth of your child demonstrates so clearly that as you increase your family you will look forward to each fresh experience and not shrink from it in fear.

Please accept my congratulations and best wishes.

Yours sincerely,
Grantly Dick Read, M.A., M.D., Cantab.

September 29, 1950

Dear Dr. Read,

I wrote you 20 months ago when our Baby G was born naturally and I absolutely could not send announcements of our Infant B without including a card to you. My doctor and I did a good job, but I know I couldn't have done it without your book. I have read it and studied it at least 4 times. In about 20 more months look for another card, I have a name for a girl I want to use, _____ _____. I hope God blesses all your efforts.

26 October 1950

Dear Mrs.,

I have received the birthday card [birth announcement] of your handsome boy. It gave me very great pleasure to know that once more you have been so clever. I wish you all happiness, and may you continue to be an apostle amongst women, and to make those who have ears and hear realize that having a baby is not just the production of a child.

If the infant arrives according to the great Design it brings with it a fuller love and bondage which not only makes homes and family units secure, but spreads its influence throughout society, which within a few generations bids fair to rid this world of the hideous turmoil which robs its peoples of so much happiness and freedom.

My best wishes to you all,

Yours very sincerely,
Grantly Dick Read, M.A., M.D., Cantab.

7 November 1951

Dear Dr. Read,

I am again the proud, happy and healthy mother of a beautiful and healthy baby girl. I must admit to being more grateful to you than ever before. Baby G was a breech birth and everything went smoothly until the last hour when she was most uncooperative about coming down. During that hour I used an ether cone to good advantage. At the end of the hour Dr. _____ decided I should discard the ether cone in favor of a needle filled with something or other. I was in full accord with him, I was awfully tired and ached all over, but being a candidate for the title of 'Most Stubborn and Cantankerous Patient in _____.' I wouldn't allow the needle unless he promised not to cut me, which I realize in the light of day was most presumptuous. However, be that as it may, I am very happy that I am such a fractious old witch for between the ether cone (which Dr. _____ knew I didn't know about because he was asleep in the doctors room) and the time consumed arguing about cutting when he came in to see what was going on, the membranes ruptured, bearing down began and I was happy again. I had beaten that needle to the punch! Hallelujah! You'll never know what that meant to me. She came cord and feet first. One nice thing about a breech, one can tell more quickly the sex, and I certainly did want a girl and I reckon I knew she was a girl a good 60 seconds sooner than I would have had she been head first.

God is so good to me, I don't see how I deserve everything I have. Here I am only 31, I have a wonderful husband who loves and indulges the lot of us more than he ever should and his is such a stimulating personality! We have the beginning of a good size family and a house large enough to meet our needs for many an additional baby. What else is there? My heart is so full of happiness today. God bless you and your family, Dr. Read. Until my next announcement.

11 January 1952

Dear Mrs.,

A late reply is better than none. Your letter gave me very great pleasure and the photograph of your children is indeed something to be proud of.

When I read the publications in American Medical Journals giving the arguments, and indeed the bland illogical statements of antagonism towards my work, I feel that the women of America should organize themselves into a great mass of apostles shouting their faith from the housetops. It is the only way that they will ever procure for themselves that which they know to be true, and which they of all people deserve.

Please convey to your husband my congratulations, and I hope that your family circle will enjoy the blessing of great happiness.

Yours very sincerely,
Grantly Dick Read, M.A., M.D., Cantab.

Correspondence 13

January 12, 1952
Washington

Dear Dr. Read,

I have read over and over your book, 'Childbirth Without Fear,' and believe that it is the greatest thing for years on obstetrics. I hope that it will be the means for many years to come of bringing joy to women in so natural a thing as childbirth—joy instead of fear, misgivings, and panic.

I had three children born while I was under the influence of drugs. Even in my ignorance of all the procedures at the hospital I had that inner feeling something was radically wrong. I had trouble nursing the last two babies and it bothered me that they were so 'dopey' that they never could be awakened when brought to nurse. I resolved that with my next baby I would be completely aware of what went on around me. Then I read parts of your book in local magazines and as a result purchased my own copy.

I couldn't begin to express in words the joy and elation that accompanied the birth of our fourth child. I believe that the medical doctor who attended me and who had been skeptical got as much thrill out of the delivery. I did not need a shot or a whiff of anything. To go a bit deeper, it was one of life's greatest spiritual experiences. To me all of the human beings in that delivery room were knit together as one with our Creator. You may understand why I look forward to having children as long as God permits.

May I express my thanks and appreciation to you for all your work and study along the lines of natural childbirth.

Very sincerely,

23 February 1952

Dear Mrs.,

It is so good of you to have written to me in the manner in which you have. I expect you realize that I get a very large number of letters from women all over the world and happily the majority of them are letters expressing gratitude for this new-found experience of Natural or Physiological Childbirth.

CMAC:PP/GDR/D.112

It is however, you ladies who have had babies the other way that are most important for it is only by the personal experience of comparison that you can really judge the complete difference between the two approaches to childbirth. You are so right in all you say and I frequently have statements from mothers who describe the birth of the child as a spiritual experience and not only a physical event. I have many letters too, from women who have told me that they had a very definite sense of a Presence in the delivery room, some one who was not of those humanly present but something or someone who brought a spirit of nearness to God at the time of the birth of their child.

I am not a parson, but at the same time I think that no obstetrician who has been present at so many natural deliveries, has witnessed the ecstasy of girls and mature women, and has heard so many of them say that this thing is nearer to the Divine than anything else they have ever experienced, cannot allow these thoughts to pass unnoticed and without a full appreciation of their significance.

What a different world we shall have when all women can feel and think as you have been led to feel and think at the birth of your child. I thank you again for writing to me so charmingly, will you please congratulate your husband on the new arrival in his family and upon the manner in which your baby has joined the flock.

My best wishes to you both,

Yours sincerely,
Grantly Dick Read, M.A., M.D., Cantab.

Correspondence 14

December 9, 1954
Herts

Dear Dr. Read,

I was surprised and delighted to hear you in 'Woman's Hour' the other day. I thought you were in the depths of the jungle, far removed from my plea for guidance!

I am 28 and have been married 8 years. During that time I have successfully avoided pregnancy, because I have always been *terrified* of the thought of childbirth pain. (I was relieved to hear, in Woman's Hour, that other women are cowards too!)

I have had nightmares, during my marriage, of becoming pregnant and going through childbirth—horrible beyond description. I have never seen a pregnant woman without thinking 'How can you look so calm when you have 'that' coming to you'. My husband knows and understands my fears so, mutually, we have taken precautions.

In August, we moved into our own house, at last, and I decided that it was 'now or never' and we must start a family before I really become too old! I could only hope my fears would diminish. (I bought your 'Revelation of Childbirth' book some two years ago &, reading that through, helped enormously in giving me a new 'slant' on childbirth, and new courage.) so I 'fell' immediately and am now about 4 months pregnant. I feel very well, and *calm* and am really looking forward to holding our baby. I do love children, in spite of this dread. My friends can't understand, (knowing me so well) why I'm not 'crawling up the wall' with nerves but perhaps one acquires some amount of placidity along with pregnancy? Nature is very clever.

I have a new doctor (new district) and he is so kind & most reassuring. This has helped me tremendously but I was rather shaken, when I asked him about relaxation classes, to hear him say 'Don't bother too much about all this relaxing business. I shall attend your confinement and you will be quite all right'! I don't agree, I know I shall panic at the end, even though I have great confidence in him.

So please, Dr. Read, will you advise me where I can attend classes on your methods and theory of relaxation so that when I face, at last, my 'nightmare' in reality I shall be ready and willing to co-operate and shall not look back on my confinement with loathing. I hope to have more than one child but it will depend on my experience whether we settle for an only child!

Is there a fairly local Centre I could attend where the staff are really *keen* and competent or would I have to come to London? Would there be fees?

I hope my letter hasn't 'rambled' too much and, whilst I appreciate how *very* busy you must be, I would be so very grateful for your advice. . . .

With sincere wishes for your success in all your good work,

Yours truly,

31 December 1954

Dear Mrs.,

Thank you for your letter of the 9th December. I have just worked down the bundle of correspondence to arrive at yours, I am sorry it has been so long unanswered.

You don't write like a woman who is frightened at fairies and who believes in old wives' stories. It seems to me that when you were a child somebody gave you some pretty poor ideas about all this business. What is really happening is that you are living on childhood assumptions that you haven't really taken the trouble to get out of your mind.

Take my advice, buy the new edition of my book and go through it carefully with your husband. . . . You will find everything there to put you straight on this matter. I cannot, of course, imagine why a healthy-minded and health-bodied[sic] woman should be frightened of having a baby. If you are properly looked after it is the most wondeful thing in the world.

I don't think much of your doctor telling you there is nothing in this relaxation business and all that. It rather sounds as if he is the sort of chap who may simply make you unconscious so that you haven't got any idea what it means to be a mother except to be a possessor of a child. I can assure you that is only about one-tenth of the real experience.

I should go round all the maternity homes and matrons of maternity hospitals in the area, spreading out within a reasonable distance of ten or fifteen miles . . . and simply ask them straight out if there is an educational class for expectant mothers. Don't only learn relaxation, you must learn your breathing and have someone tell you all about labour. If you can't find anywhere in that district at all write to me again, and I will see what I can do for you.

My best wishes,

Yours sincerely,
Grantly Dick Read, M.A., M.D., Cantab.

Correspondence 15

April 2, 1955
California

Dear Dr. Read,

. . . . I was married in 1937 when I was 22 years old. In December of 1939 I gave birth to a daughter. My memory is not too good, but I do remember being strapped down to a table, and having ether forced upon me—then nothing. The next morning I wondered why my ribs hurt—result of artificial respiration. My attending physician told me I had turned completely blue. My baby had been removed by forceps and her forehead was bruised and her head was misshapen. Of course, these conditions were outgrown. Also I was stitched inside and out, and informed by my doctor that if he ever delivered any more babies for me they would be by Cesarean section. This all took place in _____, Pennsylvania.

Following World War II, in a small town in New Mexico, August 1946, I delivered another daughter. My then attending physician was not present when I entered the hospital but the nurse on duty immediately started to give me some kind of shots. Finally I was taken to the delivery room where I was once more strapped down and forced to receive ether, (the anesthetist, a big husky man, told me later I was quite a fighter). When I came to, back to my room, the next morning I asked to see my baby, and was delighted. I learned later that she had been born blue and had to have oxygen.

Then in January 1951 I gave my first 'natural' birth! We were still living in New Mexico, but I didn't care to repeat my previous experiences so went to _____, Texas. There Dr. _____ _____ suggested I read your book and encouraged me and instructed me all during my pregnancy. I was very calm and prepared when I started in labor. There were times when I thought I might need some discomfort remover. But then Dr. _____ examined me (after only about 3 hours labor) and told me in another hour I would have my baby. So with those soothing words AND his reminder that I'd never forgive myself for not going through with natural [childbirth] we proceeded. I was wheeled into the delivery room and put on the proverbial table. I was for the third time 'put up in

---

CMAC:PP/GDR/D.109

stirrups' but they were adjusted to my comfort, and instead of my hands being strapped down I was given straps to help pull. There are many heartwarming memories for me in this delivery and since I think I have you to thank I feel inclined to tell you them. This was my first baby that only my husband and I were present. I mean none of my family. He was taking his final examinations at college earning his Bachelor of Science Degree in Civil Engineering and I had worried about missing his graduation. The baby was born on Jan. 23rd and my husband graduated on Jan. 29th, and I was there! And Dr. _____ was not only a competent physician, ordering the nurses etc. but kind to me. All the time he scrubbed he counted for me—'Push! 1, 2, 3, 4, 5, 6, 7, 8, 9, 10.' 'Take a deep breath!' etc. Then he placed a cool cloth on my forehead. And then the baby started to come and he got very busy. I will never forget the thrill when Dr. _____ held him up for me to see. And as you said Nature does anesthetize the mother. I also remember pushing out my placenta (or as we refer to it the afterbirth). The nurses were kind and considerate, but not familiar with 'natural' [childbirth]. Before I went to the delivery room one of them kept coming into the labor room with a hypodermic needle and I kept telling her I didn't want it. And in the delivery room another nurse kept offering me 'just a whiff of ether'— But after it was all over I think they were all glad to have participated. I had absolutely NO stitches as in both previous deliveries. Another innovation for me was that I could get up and walk after 24 hours after delivering. In my thank-yous I must include our monthly magazine, 'Readers' Digest' that quoted or told of your book and some of your mothers. Dr. _____ received my personal thanks and I have told any interested woman of your book.

And now for my second 'natural' birth. Following my husband's graduation we left New Mexico and came to California. And once again we were expectant parents. And as was my experience in New Mexico where I knew no doctors I inquired of my friends for a good obstetrician. I tried a few and when I asked if they'd cooperate in delivering me 'naturally' they either gave me a funny look or said that 'they did not have the time.' Now, can you imagine!! They would rather give spinals or whatever else they thought was needed. They did have the time to send the bills. Or rather the office sent the bills. Then I remembered a true DOCTOR whom I had met 10 years ago in a little town in Southern California—_____—wrote and asked him if he delivered babies he said he did and quoted his fee and from then on I was his patient. Upon my first visit I asked him if he'd help me deliver 'naturally.' His reply: 'I've delivered several thousand babies, breech, sideways, anesthesia, no anesthesia, in houses, trailers, tents and hospitals.' In other words he treated me as an intelligent woman who knew how she wanted to have her baby and also knew what she was talking about. My labor lasted a little longer this time—my cervix would not dilate—so Dr. _____ _____ ordered some kind of sedative and told the nurse to take me into the delivery room. And as soon as he said that I started to 'bear down' and Dr. _____ told me not to work so hard—to wait for a good pain—and I did. I believe he studied under Dr. _____ of Chicago. But I was not strapped down, rather informed not to touch the sterile field, and I'll never forget my relief when Dr. _____ told the nurse *not* to put me up in the stirrups! Once again I refused ether from the nurse. Several times she asked me and I kept telling her 'no' and finally Dr. _____ said: 'She's a good sport, let's go ahead.' So he gently pushed my legs down against my abdomen and from then on I don't remember too much except the nurse saying: 'There's the head!' Then Dr. _____ was awfully busy and told me I had another boy! I just wish I had thought to ask to have mirrors put up so I could have watched. Once again no stitches, and the doctor said he had never seen such a bloodless delivery. That has been almost a year ago and I still feel awed by the beautiful experience.

How can I ever thank you three! Dr. Read, Dr. _____ and Dr. _____??

I've had perfect strangers come to my door and ask me to tell them all about my 'natural' deliveries and I always recommend your books, and if they aren't already under a doctor's care, I tell them about Dr. _____. But they think that 40 miles is too far to drive. We drove that far for Dr. _____. It really took less time than to get a number, and sit with a whole bunch of other 'cattle' and wait to be called. And then get an impersonal and fast check, just like a car being run through the assembly line, or a herd being guided through the gates!

I just wish women would wise up and among us we could wise up the medical profession. After all, we're the ones who have the babies! Just a little education and guidance is all we need. I didn't even know where my uterus was until Dr. _____ showed me.

Dr. Read, you can feel that your books are like pebbles tossed into a pool and I for one am helping to increase the size to the circles you have made. I just wish Dr. _____ and Dr. _____ would have the time to write some books too.

And now would you answer a question for me: What does 'Cantab., Stoner House, Steep, Nr. Petersfield, Hants,' all mean?

Yours most gratefully,

7th May 1955

Dear Mrs.,

I feel ashamed that your letter should have been in my study for three weeks and not yet replied to, but it is infrequently that I receive a letter that has given me so much pleasure and pride to read.

It really is grand to hear, and happily I do frequently hear, of medical men who have got the humanity and good sense to assist their patients to have their babies without unnecessary interference and what I call meddlesome nonsense, which is so frequently thought to be modern science.

The story of your first two labors, which unhappily I hear all too often from the United States is one which should be published all over the world and then should be followed by your reactions to the second two labors. I think there can be no greater weight of persuasion than the history of the arrival of the family of a woman like yourself. Perhaps that does throw rather a big responsibility on you when I say that because it is ladies like yourself who definitely can do so much good in the world even though it is against the modern training of some of the medical schools.

Fortunately as I expect you realize, this very natural approach to childbirth although it has got many names in America, is spreading rapidly and I do believe in good time the American women will have just exactly what they deserve for their common sense. I might add, by the way, that my wife is half-American prompts me to write like this.

I do wish you could see a film I took of the last four cases I delivered before I left South Africa. It is the most perfect example of women as they should behave having their babies naturally, and the enjoyment, the whole happiness of the proceedings although three out of them could not be described as absolutely normal in some ways. It is worth seeing. I am trying to get the distributors to make it available in America for those who would like to have and show it to women who need the sort of help of which they are so well aware.

All I can say is thank you very much indeed for writing me so fully, I appreciate it a lot, and I hope you won't mind if I use your letter sometimes without using your name. I have got many hundreds of which I have asked that question and from time to time one or the other seems to be very fitting for the occasion. You also enquire 'What is Cantab.?' Cantab. is the short for Cambridge and indicates my University. When my name is signed M.A., M.D., Cantab. it means I got those two degrees at Cambridge University.

Stoner House is the name of my house which is built on the hillside of the Stoner Ridge, in a village by the name of Steep, and that is about two miles from a small market town named Petersfield in the county of Hampshire. Well, you see we have cut it down very short haven't we, but happily your letter reached me safely.

I am going to write to Drs. _____ and _____ because I do like to get in touch with men like that. So many women write and ask me if they can be given the names of a doctor who will help them have their baby as I teach it. My list grows, and I would like to write and ask these two men whether their names can be put on that list.

My best wishes to you and please congratulate your husband on having you for a wife, and I must say I also congratulate your children particularly the last two without any difference in feeling but they have been born as I believe the Creator intended they should.

Yours very sincerely,
Grantly Dick Read, M.A., M.D., Cantab.

Correspondence 16

October 26, 1955
Kentucky

Dear Dr. Read,

I am writing this to thank you for your deep understanding about childbirth. With the help of your wonderful book, 'Childbirth Without Fear,' my husband and I experienced the most glorious moment of our lives. Our son was born naturally.

After the birth of our little daughter three and a half years ago, I felt I would never have another child if I had to go through that horrible experience of labor again. I will not go into details except that I had the usual delivery; my husband and I were separated and I was drugged. Even then I knew that birth should not have been the nightmare it was.

As time passed I felt a deep desire for another child. Finally I found a doctor and hospital that truly understood the needs of a pregnant woman. Now I know there is nothing on earth to equal the thrill and holiness of feeling and seeing and hearing one's own child born. My husband was by my side during labor and delivery, and my baby was by my side during my stay in the hospital. Now I pray that I will be blessed with many more children.

Dr. Read, your book is truth, and I cannot understand why every woman and doctor will not open their eyes to this truth. If ever I can help you in your great work, please notify me. I am very interested in educating the public about natural childbirth. Recently I have met many women who have bore[sic] their babies naturally after reading your book. Perhaps they did not sit down and write you a letter, but I know they are grateful to you.

Dr. Read, I wanted desperately to nurse my babies, but was unable to. I did not seem to be able to satisfy their appetites. If you can give me any advice, I would appreciate it so very much.

Sincerely,

3 November 1955

Dear Mrs.,

Thank you for your letter of the 26th October. I was most grateful to receive it and I do congratulate you sincerely on having, through the

CMAC:PP/GDR/D.116

birth of your second baby, appreciated what the Creator intended the birth of your baby to be like.

You write so much that I agree with and I never cease to wonder why so many members of my profession refuse to pay any attention whatever to this wonderful experience women can have if they are helped in the proper way.

I was extremely interested that you had a doctor who was able to assist you in this. Would you like to tell me what hospital and who the doctor is, because I do get a large number of women who write to me about this and where they can find a doctor, some even say anywhere in the United States, and others may within a hundred miles and so on. It would be a great help to many people if I knew that.

You ask me how you can help in this work. May I tell you that your sentence is probably the best of all helps and that is, 'Your book is truth,'; you could add, I have tried without it and I have tried with it, and I understand the difference.

I think your inability to feed the baby probably arises from some complex which occurred when the first baby was coming or at its arrival. I am quite sure that anyone who can enjoy the birth of their second child as you have, should be physically able to feed the baby. I don't know whether you believe in measures like hypnosis, but a friend of mine in Chicago has brought the milk back into a mother's breasts enabling her to feed her baby simply by correcting something that has arisen in the mind through a past and unpleasant experience.

Now this is only a suggestion, because naturally I don't know your circumstances or where you live, but that is a suggestion. Other than that, a little warm massage of the breast, drink plenty of milk and plenty of water and at the same time get completely relaxed when you are feeding your baby, and allow your baby to do the rest.

My best wishes to you, and I do hope all goes well with you.

Yours sincerely,
Grantly Dick Read, M.A., M.D., Cantab.

December 10, 1955

Dear Dr. Read,

I was delighted to receive your letter. I am not very good at putting into words what I feel in my heart, but I do hope my letter gave you some idea of how very much your teachings have helped me. Again I ask you to call upon me if ever I can be of assistance.

The name of my doctor is Dr. _____. His office is in _____. Dr.

_____ of _____ also encourages natural childbirth. The hospital is _____ _____ Hospital. Both _____ and _____ are suburbs of Louisville, Kentucky.

Not a single hospital in Louisville permits the father in the labor or delivery room. None have private labor rooms. Nor do they permit the child to room with its mother. They actually discourage breast feeding as the baby is permitted to remain with its mother only about ten minutes, four times a day. If the baby does not nurse during the allotted period, it is given a bottle. The rules completely refuse to allow the awakening of mothers for the night feeding. Many mothers are not even allowed to see their child (except through the glass nursery window) for over a twenty-four hour period. In this time of modern hospitals, it is almost unbelievable that better facilities are not available on the maternity wards. It seems we women have for years been propagandized with fear and hospital rules. Many would rather fall into the pits of twilight sleep than put out effort and 'bear down.' Yet many more would break this custom if only an understanding doctor and hospital were available. I think it is time for women to rebel!

_____ _____ Hospital is small, and not so modern as compared to the new ultra-modern hospitals in Louisville, but to me it offers a great deal more. Dr. _____ and Dr. _____ are general practitioners, but they are much more understanding to the ways of a pregnant woman than are any of the obstetricians in Louisville. Only one obstetrician in Louisville permits natural childbirth. He is Dr. _____, but the hospitals will not permit the presence of the father or rooming-in. It is even almost impossible to find a doctor to assist in a prearranged home delivery. It seems a shame to punish the women who are not afraid to bear their children naturally because of the women who are afraid.

If you would let me know the name of the doctor in Chicago, if ever I were in Chicago, I could make an appointment with him. Thank you again for taking the time to answer my last letter. It was much appreciated. I wish you a very Merry Christmas and successful New Year.

                                                                Sincerely,

23 December 1955

Dear Mrs.,

It was very nice to hear from you and you sent me a letter of very considerable assistance. I agree with every word you have said. Why healthy, happy women should have to suffer the routine of treatment for those who are neither healthy nor happy is quite unforgivable in modern civilization, but it goes on although we must really agree, I think, that the effort made to change things is becoming more and more important.

If you visit Chicago at any time, I think you would enjoy calling upon Dr. _____ and telling him that you followed out my procedures and explain to him what went on in the hospital. I am sure he would be interested.

In the meantime, do settle down to a really happy and healthy New Year. In this country, the wisest decision is so often to take the advice of your general practitioner, have your baby at home and be cared for under his observation.

I am quite sure you would not regret it and it would at least isolate you from the influences you have described.

My best wishes to you,

Yours sincerely,
Grantly Dick Read, M.A., M.D., Cantab.

Correspondence 17

23 January 1956
Lewisham

Dear Dr. Read,

After reading your article, 'Children Without Pain,' I too long to have my second baby, due in August by the same method.

Many times since my first child was born I have felt that I didn't enjoy his birth to the full. Though until now, never realized why. Due to ignorance and fear I suffered a great deal of pain during my eleven hours of labour. Not helped by a remark from a sister. 'Don't pull faces like that, you have a lot worse to come.' I was given drugs to help me to relax. So that by the time my baby was born though I was conscious, my brain was dulled by the drugs and I did not fully appreciate the wonderful achievement of birth.

Another thing that my husband and I have discussed a great deal and agree upon is that he should be present when our baby is born. Not only do I feel that he should share the joy and fulfillment but that I should gain reassurance and happiness by his presence.

Please can you advise me what to do, and is there any literature we can read, to help us understand and enjoy the coming of our second child?

Yours sincerely,

15 February 1956

Dear Mrs.,

Thank you very much for your letter of January 23. . . .

You do not say whether you are going to have this baby at home or in the hospital, or whether you have arranged to attend any antenatal classes.

I would suggest that you get my book, 'Childbirth Without Fear,' and read this thoroughly, and then if you have any further queries, write to me again. Another little book you will find most useful is 'Antenatal Illustrated' which has only just been published and costs 3/6d. This sets out briefly the principles of natural childbirth and is an easy reference

---

CMAC:PP/GDR/D.46

for breathing, relaxation and a few exercises, but for greater detail you would need the larger book for reference.

  With best wishes,

Yours sincerely.
Grantly Dick Read, M.A., M.D., Cantab.

Section 4

Twentieth Century
Patient/Physician Relationship by Mail

*"Please forgive me troubling you when you must be very
busy but I would be extremely gratified for some advice."*

This section illustrates women's need for a physician, and, consequently, women in Britain and the United States wrote to Dick-Read
asking for advice on their pregnancies and labors. Some women were
looking for a referral to a physician who practiced Dick-Read's methods, while others were seeking his opinions on the medical aspects of
their pregnancies. But unlike in other sections there was a level of ex-
pectation in these letters for a response from Dick-Read. Since he wrote
the instructions for health during pregnancy and how women should
conduct themselves in labor, women felt he was "their" doctor and that
he would help them. For his part, Dick-Read did not disappoint the
women who wrote to him. He assumed the role of "physician-by-mail."
We learn of Dick-Read's disapproval of the routine interference with
childbirth by his American colleagues and his suggestions that it was
something stressed as part of the American medical education. Finally,
Dick-Read's clear insights on the role of women in the post-war societies of England and the United States are highlighted in the correspondence that follows.

Correspondence 18

April 14, 1947
Illinois

Dear Dr. Read:

I have just recently completed your book, 'Childbirth Without Fear.' Before reading it, I had many notions about natural childbirth very similar to the theory you express, but never before had I heard it expressed so clearly and backed up so factually by a professional man. I wanted to write you to tell you how enthusiastic I am about your progress, and how much I hope you will be able to continue your work and train students along the lines of your theories.

I also wanted to write you to ask you to do me a favor—if it is within your power. If I were in England, without hesitation I should make every effort to become a patient of yours when my second baby arrives next October. Here in America, in _____, I have been making fruitless investigations to find a male or female physician who believes in natural childbirth. So far all that I have traced believe in the use of analgesics— especially Nembutal—and anesthetics, at least nitrous oxide. Part of the reason for the anesthetic use seems to be the routine episiotomy. I have been unable to find any physician who believed in educating a mother to deliver the baby *herself* and who cared about developing expert skills preventing tears rather than in perfecting the surgical techniques of episiotomies.

I happen to have been a medical student—I attended the _____ Medical School here in _____ for almost three years, and I hope to finish my M.D. degree eventually, when my family is completed. This is another reason why I have been interested, all along, in the methods of obstetrics.

My first baby was delivered by the navy clinic (she is now 16 months old). I had nothing to say about the conduct of labor, of course, and I didn't even know what doctor was to assist me until I was in labor. Luckily I knew enough about the mechanics of labor to help myself a good bit; and I believe fear was reduced considerably. Also, I was lucky enough to have a calm and steadfast husband by my side throughout the first stage of labor. However, I was routinely given Nembutal (which seemed to precipitate the second stage), and I was completely under an anesthetic after the head started coming through (although I was

CMAC:PP/GDR/D.110

allowed to see my baby right after she was born). In the course of delivery my cervix was badly torn. No instruments were used—the baby was large (8 pounds 6 ounces); I do not know why the cervix was torn unless it was because I did not relax at the right times. According to my physician, I cooperated very well with what instructions he gave me.

Now, the favor I want to ask of you is this: do you know of any physician in the Chicago area, or elsewhere in the United States who is in sympathy with your views and practices them? Even if such a man were far away from Chicago, if you could give me his name and address I could write him and ask him to recommend a Chicago physician.

I cannot tell you how grateful I will be for any assistance you can give me in finding a physician who believes in natural childbirth.

Again, may I wish you the greatest success in your work and may I urge you to write more books about it and especially to include more of those excellent case histories.

Sincerely,

23rd April 1947

Dear Mrs.,

Thank you for your very interesting letter. I hope I can be of some help to you.

When I was in Chicago in February I met most of the obstetricians there. It seemed to me that the practice of physiological childbirth is not, at present, carried out with a very full measure of interest at the Lying-In Hospital but at the Maternity Center Association at Chicago which was started by Dr. _____ _____ many years ago, his nephew, _____ _____, practices from time to time. There is also an excellent woman doctor there of whom I took a very good view from the point of view of her work and a man who was also very good but I regret to tell you I cannot remember his name. The experience and the outlook of the Chicago Maternity Center is probably very much more in keeping with what you desire than the more academic outlook at the Lying-In Hospital. I suggest that you get in touch with either the woman whose name I can't remember or Dr. _____ _____, tell them that you want your baby in the manner that I advise and what can they do about it to help you to obtain these measures.

If you have any difficulty there I have sent a copy of your letter (I hope not presumptuously) to Miss Hazel Corbin of the Maternity Center Association, 654 Madison Avenue, New York, because they are in full sympathy with these procedures and I send to them a large number of letters that I receive from American ladies who ask me exactly the same thing that you have done. I am sure Miss Corbin will give you every help and she does know the people who are conducting child-birth in this way. It makes having babies so easy and so happy and establishes such a sense of achievement in a mother's mind that the demand for this is rapidly spreading all over the world.

I am sitting in my library at the sunrise of a beautiful English spring morning at my country house about twenty miles from London. I have just returned from delivering a woman of thirty-two of her first child. She was a dour, undemonstrative sort of person and was not persuaded that my teaching was applicable to her; she, like so many other women, felt that she really was rather different from other people. Her first baby weighed well over 7 lbs, from beginning to end it took ten hours, she sat up and watched it born and looked at me rather superiorily and said 'But this is ridiculous—hold it up a little higher Doctor, are you sure it is a girl? Ah, it is, dear, dear, we had hoped for a boy but still, this is very wonderful and I am more than pleased.' (They had hoped for a boy because they happen to have a good deal of this world's goods) but just to give you that as an example. I feel that anyone who writes to me is a personal friend of mine or they wouldn't do it.

Write and let me know if you have any luck in getting hold of the right people to do this. It's your heritage to have your baby as you want and if you have already had an 8lb. 6oz. child I am perfectly certain that you can have your next one physiologically if you get adequate assistance and education.

Yours sincerely,
Grantly Dick Read, M.A., M.D., Cantab.

Correspondence 19

19 October 1950
London

Dear Dr. Grantly Dick Read,
   Please forgive my troubling you when you must be very busy, but I would be extremely gratified for some advice.
   I am 25 years of age and expect my first baby in the first week of June 1951. I heard of your methods of Natural Childbirth some years ago and was very impressed. I decided then that, should I ever have any children, I should do all in my power to follow your methods. As soon as I thought I might be pregnant my husband and I bought. . . your book, 'Childbirth Without Fear,' which I have now read.
   I intend having my baby in London but, not knowing anyone who has followed your teaching, I am at a loss to know which doctor, or which clinic to go to for antenatal care. I realize from your book that, should I be unlucky in my choice of doctor, I may meet some opposition—or, at any rate, some skepticism. At the birth, too, I might have unwanted analgesia forced upon me. I feel quite sure there must be many antenatal Clinics in London which now believe in your teachings and, could I be under their care, I should be quite happy.
   My husband is an actor so that our finances are very uncertain and I shall have to work until a few weeks before the baby arrives. I am not registered with any London doctor as we have been moving round the countryside until now. However, my husband has recently had the offer of a London job and we shall be resident in London, at the above address from now on.
   Once again I do apologize for troubling you, but your book has given me such confidence and there is no-one else who can give me advice upon this matter.

Yours sincerely,

P.S. Stamped, addressed envelope enclosed.

CMAC:PP/GDR/D.43

13 November 1950

Dear Mrs.,

Thank you for your letter. I am afraid it has taken rather a long time to arrive.

May I strongly advise you to go to _____ Hospital and ask to see Professor _____ if he is there (I know he has recently been in America), or his second in command. The address is _____ Hospital. . . .

From that source I am sure you will get every assistance, and it may be possible even that you are admitted to either the public or private rooms of _____ Hospital, according to the size of your purse. I am not certain of the organization of the London Hospitals under the new Health Service, but I am confident that this advise will give you an opportunity of receiving ante-natal and natal care along the line that I teach.

My best wishes.

Yours sincerely,
Grantly Dick Read, M.A., M.D., Cantab.

2 February 1952

Dear Dr. Grantly Dick Read,

This is a most belated letter to say thank-you for some advice you gave me about where I should have my baby in London so that I could follow your methods of antenatal preparation. You advised me to go to Professor _____ of _____ Hospital, but as it happened, when your letter arrived I had already booked at _____ Hospital as time was getting on. I know you will be interested to know that _____ Hospital works entirely upon your methods. There are weekly 'classes' for the expectant mothers where the exercises and relaxation are taught, and there are regular lectures as well. I could not have asked more!

I worked up until six weeks before my baby was expected but managed to exercise and relax each day nevertheless. I felt very well all the time and had no complaints whatsoever. The actual birth was all that you say it should be and was indeed the most wonderful and satisfying experience I have ever had. I was offered analgesia but would not be bothered with it. I was in labour for 56 1/2 hours but, apart from feeling extremely impatient, I had no complaints. I was in a large ward and I think you will be amused to know that from 5 am onwards (the baby was born at 7 am) on the morning of the birth I kept my poor neighbors awake by repeating every five minutes 'Remember to relax—relax your right leg—relax your left leg'—and so on. I had no idea that I was saying these things aloud. I knew I was thinking them hard every time I felt a contraction coming but I seemed to be quite be-mused. I fell fast asleep, in any case, between contractions. As a matter of fact I had been sleeping so well that I found it difficult to convince the nurses that I was in the second stage when it came at 6 am. I remember feeling most hurt and hard-done-by at the time! Incidentally, in the ordinary way I should have been moved out of the general ward before this but that night there were five other births and only a mid-wife, medical student and two nurses on duty so that they were very busy.

I needed no stitches and was allowed to see the after-birth as I requested and was duly amazed! As I was being wheeled back into the ward the sister thanked me for being 'so co-operative.' I told her that it wasn't me she should thank but you. And she heartily agreed!

I do thank you most sincerely. I had practically memorized your book and never once did anything happen which I was not prepared for and that was the greatest help of all—that, and not being afraid.

Yours very sincerely and gratefully,

PS. The baby was a boy and weighed 7 1/2 lbs. He is now seven months old and weighs 20 1/2 lbs and is fine!

23 February 1952

Dear Mrs.,

I was delighted to receive your letter and once or twice had rather wondered what had happened to you. It was very kind of you to write so fully about your labour and I do congratulate you that you were able to carry out the procedures of my teaching so well.

I had no idea that _____ Hospital had really got down to this work; you see, I am the last person in the world that the members of the staff of the big hospitals communicate with when they are using my procedures. Directly I got your letter I wrote a note to Mr. _____ asking him how it was all going and whether he thought it was worth while. I expect he will write to me soon because I know him quite well.

This is the fifth letter this evening that I have replied to who tells me much the same delightful story that you have written in your letter. I can only congratulate you and tell you how very much this will bring to you in the future, not only the satisfaction of the immediate achievement, but you will notice the manner in which he adjusts himself to the changing phases of life. I think further you will notice an astonishing sense of close mother-child relationship; he will always be of you so long as you allow, and so long as you follow the natural maternal instinct and eschew the teaching of the modern, scientific pediatrician. I would not for one moment cast any aspersion upon those whose learning is greater than their experience, but I am persuaded that no one understands motherhood better than an intelligent mother and no child really seeks advice and leadership of anyone other than his mother.

Yours sincerely,
Grantly Dick Read, M.A., M.D., Cantab.

Correspondence 20

24 September 1951
Kent

Dear Dr. Dick Read,
    Having just read your book, my husband and I are very keen to get some advice from you. . . .
    We feel very strongly that your method is right and the only reasonable and sensible way to give birth to children. However, believing is one thing and carrying it out another, and this is where I badly need help.
    So far, we have not started a child, and don't wish to until we are able to follow advice from a doctor or midwife who is in sympathy with your method (preferably one who knows about it and shows the relaxation exercises etc rather than one who lets you practise what you like but is not much more than an onlooker.)
    We live in a two roomed flat, with kitchen and bathroom, so for these days, we cannot be said to be badly off. I do part time teaching in the flat (private piano pupils) and I am hoping that I can continue this through pregnancy, and after the child is born. I am very interested in my work, and felt that it was one of the few things that one could do without in any way upsetting the upbringing of the child. I should, however, be glad to know if you agree with this!
    Nowadays, I think most people take advantage of the Health Service, and, in fact we ourselves would be crippled without it. So the first difficulty is for us to find somebody we can really trust, for our doctor. So far, I have only been to the doctor with whom we registered once during the two years we have been here, and that for a trivial thing. My husband has been several times, and we neither of us found much satisfaction from our visits, and myself, I don't feel I want him to attend me during pregnancy. It is not easy to know which is the best doctor to go to, but I am quite certain that if there were a doctor here who followed your methods I should feel safe and confident that any queries and doubts on my part would be cleared up sympathetically. On the other hand, if I were to have the baby at *home*, then a midwife with all the same methods as mentioned above, should be perfect.
    My husband and I feel that the ideal thing is to have the baby at home, and we decided that, given a person we both trusted, and pro-

CMAC:PP/GDR/D.38

vided everything was all set for a normal birth, then he would like to have felt to have been some use. To my mind, the First Stage seems the obvious time, as you mention one needs company perhaps, and though it might be desirable that a doctor or midwife should be with one throughout labour, these days I am certain that it does not happen. We feel that if I can be taught about relaxation and about the working of my body during pregnancy and labour (I know very little about it, and your book had many surprises for me, and much that I still am not certain of, not knowing the medical terms), and of course, if I relay all that I am being taught, to my husband, then we should be able to manage very well by ourselves, here, with professional help at the end.

After much explanation on my part I feel sure you would like me to state just exactly what information I require. It is this: do you happen to know of a doctor or midwife under whom I can register (when we do manage to conceive a child) who will instruct me in your teachings? Quite possibly you have no record of any who use your method, in which case I wonder, if others write to you for the same advice, stating they can't do anything privately, what advice you are able to give them? I shall be pleased to hear of anything that will give me hope that we shall be able to have what we want. Perhaps there is a clinic attached to one of the London hospitals, that caters for information thirsty people! I thought I had heard of a place that gave instruction during pregnancy, but whether it has just information or whether there were definite relaxing lessons etc, and, which hospital it was I don't know.

I do know that I am too ignorant still, to carry out your suggestions in a hospital, or with a doctor who is sympathetic or even against the principles and tries to give an anaesthetic. I had a friend who wanted to have a natural birth, who had read your book, and was managing on her own, but during labour, the staff of a hospital at _____ were dreadful to her. She had two injections, against her wish, which made her half doped throughout the proceedings, and unable to protest at the way things were carried out. She did manage I believe without anaesthetic, and told us it was altogether a grand experience, but she had strength of mind to withstand opposition, and I feel I know myself well enough to say that I doubt being able to do that, without having had very careful teaching before hand, to be able to defy nurses and others who do stupid and unnecessary things for one.

If you could tell me your correct fee I should, more than anything love to make just one appointment with you for a general talk, or, possibly, be able to do a certain amount through a few postal talks, but this would have to be just a luxury on my part, extra to help from whoever I am registered for the birth on the National Health Service scheme.

This is very anticipatory of me, I feel, as I believe often, if one wants a child too much, it is sometimes not possible to have one for sometime, especially if one uses a contraceptive, as we do at the moment. Also, I hope it is not a very cold blooded way of going about this, but we want to have the baby when (a) it is most convenient for me to possibly cancel some teaching for a month or two, (b) when my husband is at home most to help, and (c) when we can both be free to enjoy the experience and have a month or so to get into the new routine. We both teach, and therefore, have the two month holiday in the summer, so, we want to have the baby in July, August, or September of next year. The middle month is the ideal one, but I feel we must be as elastic as possible, or no baby, will be the result, and it might mean waiting another year for which I should be very sorry.

I have no more queries that I can ask now, until I hear your good, or bad news. I enclose a small fee. Though I feel sure it doesnt [sic] cover what you really charge, I should be glad to send more as soon as you let me know the exact amount. I do feel that this is as good as any consultation, and should therefore be treated as such. If for any reason you dont [sic] accept enquiries by post or for any reason cannot take the cheque, I would rather it went into some research funds [for] something in which you are interested, rather than have it returned to me, I am sure you will do that.

Thank you so much in anticipation of your reply, I feel already, having got this long letter off my chest, that thing[s] are going to turn out well for us. (If you recommend any other books to read by you or another author, I should be grateful for their names.)

With best wishes,

Yours sincerely,

I enclose a stamped addressed envelope for reply.

17 October 1951

Dear Mrs.,

You will see from my address that it is not easy for you to meet me to discuss this matter personally, but I can most certainly give you advice that can be helpful to you.

I would like you to study carefully my book 'Introduction to Motherhood' after having read 'Childbirth without Fear', which will give you a close insight into both the theory and practice of Physiological Childbirth.

Many women from the most outlandish corners of the earth have written to me saying that they have been completely successful through the help of the husbands in having their babies at home with the minimum of discomfort, attended only by a nurse who had very little knowledge previously of the technique. You will probably do much better with a good midwife and a doctor on call if necessary than have a doctor who has neither sympathy with nor understanding of this approach to childbirth.

I have lectured in Maidstone and in Canterbury on more than one occasion, and I suggest that you go to the hospitals and enquire of the matron in charge of Obstetrics whether there are doctors on their staff who are practising my procedures, and secondly you should enquire whether there are any organized ante-natal schools.

At one or other of these two cities there is a modern Obstetrics hospital, but unfortunately I cannot remember which it is although I think it is Canterbury. From the hospital that I have in mind a report was published upon their work in Natural Childbirth, written I believe by women doctors.

These enquiries are more than likely to bring you the necessary assistance; if, however, they should not prove fruitful, then write to Prof. _____, of _____ Hospital, London, who is to a certain extent utilising this method, and he may be able to advise you upon the correct course to take.

It is very kind of you to forward to me £2.2-, and I can assure you that if all the hundreds of enquiries who write to me did the same, a considerable sum could be set aside to be devoted to the expenses of the Ante-Natal School in this town, which is doing wonderful work, but which unfortunately has to be run at a considerable financial loss. It is to this end that your cheque will be utilised.

My best wishes,

Yours sincerely,
Grantly Dick Read, M.A., M.D., Cantab.

Correspondence 21

January 18, 1952
Washington

Dear Dr. Read,

I am presuming a great deal in writing to you—presuming that you will receive and read this and not consider it a complete waste of your time. However, I have just read your book, Childbirth Without Fear, and it impressed me as being the message of a sincere and perhaps inspired man seeking the fulfillment of a very noble ideal. If this is true then I would like to add to your success the knowledge of one more convert.

Your theories and principles appeared to be very new, but I noticed your book was published eight years ago and I'm sure has gained wide acceptance since then. Yet of course, the practicing obstetricians of today would be the last to become convinced. However, a theory so simple and fundamentally true must become recognized. To me it was a story that was a joy to hear because it only reinforced what I instinctively feel to be true. Of course, I have heard all kinds of stories in the course of my development, and I accepted pain and difficulty as the natural accompaniments of birth simply because I was in no position to possess or investigate the facts. I have a curious turn of mind and have made it my business to find out as much as possible concerning the circumstances of reproduction ever since I was a child. Luckily I have a mother who discussed freely and with pride the circumstances of the birth of her children though she unfortunately went through the usual procedure of gas and stitches.

I am 22 years old and have recently graduated from college and now find myself a housewife and mother-to-be. Recently a good friend of mine underwent the birth of her third child according to the principles of your method of natural childbirth which her doctor had found very successful. She, of course, was an enthusiastic convert after comparing the results of the last birth with the preceding painful ones. Both the mother and the baby recovered in splendid condition and she claims that she was so excited and stimulated by it all that she couldn't go to sleep after the baby had arrived. Evidence like that is hard to disbelieve.

I myself believe I am in perfect biological condition to have my baby and am determined that it shall be an experience which is thrilling to

CMAC:PP/GDR/D.105

recall. I have always felt that I am perfectly fitted to give birth and am delighted that I am soon to have my own baby. However when I found I was pregnant I waited till my third month and then went to an obstetrician who I had heard highly recommended from several different sources. I told him that I wanted to have my baby according to the principles of the Read method, natural childbirth. He treated this with a 'Dr. knows best' attitude and told me that childbirth without anesthesia was cruel and inhumane. I was naturally confused by this opinion from a man who was obviously a very efficient and successful doctor, so I said no more about it. Now I can understand that he is kind and capable in his own way and only does his best to relieve the suffering he witnesses. I would like to find a doctor who believes in natural childbirth, but I don't know where to go, and the thought occurred to me that perhaps I could be a living example to this doctor. Now this is rather an ambitious project for an ignorant girl to pursue, yet after reading your book and absorbing the ideas as near to first hand as possible, I feel convinced that I could do it if my moral stamina holds up. I don't have anyone to teach me how to relax or tell me if I'm doing it all right. I have no one to support my plan when I have misgivings, no one to lean on for advice, etc. I am going to try. Everything is so clear to me that I'm sure I can't be afraid if everything goes normally. I will learn how to relax as I go and depend upon my calm and understanding husband for moral support if necessary.

I felt impelled to write to you because I wanted to assure you that your theory was spreading and that you would certainly live to see widespread acceptance and success. However, this must certainly have already come to pass and my encouragement is unnecessary; but just the same it is so important and revolutionary to me that I had to let you know. Perhaps you can see for yourself that each success is like a pebble dropped in a pool which spreads knowledge and truth with each widening ripple. And now it is affecting your neighbors across the ocean. This is only one small testimony of the courage you have given so many mothers to have confidence in their own natural abilities.

I would give anything to be able to benefit from your care or even to talk to you, but since this is impossible I must be content with the knowledge you have provided. You probably get dozens of such letters everyday. But, just in case this experiment of mine isn't too usual and captures your interest, I would be delighted to tell you how I come out of it if you want to go to the trouble of having someone drop me a card. I would like to tell you all kinds of things that differentiate my pregnancy from all others—the fact that I may have twins if our original schedule of arrival on May 22 is correct. I felt life December 9 which put me a month ahead of myself. And at 4 months I measured big enough to be 6 months along. Then, I have heart trouble (the effects of rheumatic fever or a congenital condition.) But enough of that.

I wish I could express the gratitude I feel for the new confidence and clarity of vision I find are mine due directly to your efforts. I only hope for the control to prove you right.

I remain in your debt,

10 March 1952

Dear Mrs.,

I was delighted to receive your interesting and enthusiastic letter. May I offer just a word of simple advice as from a friend and not from a medical man.

There are women all over the world today who are having their babies naturally in spite of their medical attendants, a large number of whom are still skeptical or ignorant of these procedures.

If you have not got a small book of mine called 'Introduction to Motherhood', you should obtain a copy without delay, for you will find in it a good deal of practical instruction on your [sic] to assist yourself. The three great virtues of a woman in labor are self-control, patience and the ability to work hard without any fear once the bearing down of the second stage is established.

You will find upon a close examination of your sensations that the majority of your discomforts will be threatening discomforts rather than a real thing. Labor is a test of a woman's character, and thus if you have courage and perseverance, and providing your medical man can assure you that the position of your child and the relative size of the baby to the birth canal are satisfactory, your uterus will present you with a baby if you will give it a chance and not interfere with its action by the anticipation of discomfort, and if you remain relaxed and patient.

You might, at the transition from the first to the second stage experience some back ache but this goes shortly after your expulsive efforts start. You may, when the head stretches the ultimate outlet of the birth canal, experience a sensation of burning with a threatening of bursting. These things will not occur if you desist from making too great an effort as the baby's head is ready to be born; breathe rapidly without pushing and your baby will be extruded by the uterus with the least possible difficulty. Bear these things in mind for they are friendly advice from a stranger who has appreciated your letter.

As you say quite rightly, I receive a vast number of letters from all over the world in languages I cannot understand and that have to be translated for me. Yours however, is beautifully compiled, a simple straightforward expression of your feelings and desires. Let me give you, therefore, my sincere good wishes for courage and perseverance for these two combined with the understanding of which you are obviously capable, you will be able to achieve your wishes. Be kind to your doctor when he wants to interfere but tell him that you prefer to go on as you are confident that all will be well.

My kind regards,

Yours sincerely,
Grantly Dick Read, M.A., M.D., Cantab.

Correspondence 22

July 11, 1952
Ohio

My dear Dr. Read,

It is my sincere hope that this letter with its meager address should find its way to you.

On June 13 I had my first child (6lbs., 8oz.) and followed your method as closely as any lay-person could. Our family doctor also agreed to assist me in this venture. In view of the size and extremely favorable position of the baby.

However, the general attitude in the greater _____, Ohio, area seems to be that 'Read is O.K., but he goes too far.' This brings to mind one or two questions that I find unanswered in your book 'Childbirth Without Fear.' After I had dilated about 1/2 inch, I was given instructions to strain the sphincter muscles with each successive contraction while the doctor and my husband took turns pushing on my knees. This I continued to do for almost two hours before being taken to the delivery room.

Since the contractions during this time were about 30 to 40 seconds apart, I was quite exhausted.

After being taken to the delivery room, my wrists were strapped down and my legs strapped to metal stirrups and I was told to pull upward and outward on metal handles and to continue straining the sphincter muscles. After 1/2 hour of this I could feel the baby's head ease up to the opening and then I remembered to relax.

Just prior to this stage, I had to be catharized—an extremely painful process. Fortunately, it was the only pain I had experienced with the exception of the usual enema and a couple of rough rectal examinations in the beginning.

For several minutes after I had felt the head I was aware of only a dreamy satisfaction during which, my husband tells me, I babbled on about pulling weeds and planting radishes. I remember doing a very thick-tongued job of trying to tell a joke I had heard the day before. Also, during this period, the doctor was pushing the head back from the opening and easing it forward again. The next thing I felt was the emergence of the head, turning as it came. This was so very unexpected that I screamed, knowing I would pull in and tear as I did so.

Thoroughly angry, I screamed once more as I felt the baby being pulled out, figuring that the damage had already been done and that I was entitled to a little show of temper. The resultant pain ceased at once and the afterbirth was expelled comfortably with very little bleeding.

I confirmed the necessity of stitches with the doctor and settled back in relief only to be jarred half silly when he began tucking in a fairly large hemorrhoid. Expecting more of the same, I jumped around when he began prodding the perineum to determine the extent of the tear. Then came the business of a sort of whip-stitching the vulva which hurt a little each time he pulled up the thread to see where he was going. I yapped good-naturedly about it and we were through.

The point of my letter is this—we did the best we could, but I feel that the prolonged straining of the sphincter was not only tiring but unnecessary. I have always had regular movements and the small skin flaps around the rectum have hindered my recovery considerably since the menstrual flow seemed to start up again if I went more than twelve hours without a movement.

I don't intend to start another child until this rectal condition is completely abated. I seriously doubt that I will ever start another if forced to go through several hours of straining 'to make the baby come faster.' In your case histories I can find no reference to this straining in order to speed up dilation of the cervix and would appreciate your comment on its necessity. Am making a copy of this letter should you desire that it be shown to our doctor with your reply.

Dr. Read, I appreciate the importance of your time and would be most eager to comply with any conditions contingent upon your reply. We'd like two more children, so this is most important to us.

Sincerely yours,

P.S.   Age 27—Primipara
        Height: 5'6"
        Weight at Conception: 109 lbs.
        Weight prior to birth: 131 lbs
        Weight two weeks later: 112 1/2 lbs
        Time of conception: Sept. 18, 1951
        Length of pregnancy: 38 weeks and two days
        Complications due to pregnancy: None
        Complications during pregnancy: Spontaneous Pneumothorax
           during third month resulting in terrific mental strain and
           discontinuance of exercises until February 1, 1952. Lung

went down to25% of capacity November 19 and showed
complete re-expansion in fluoroscope about December 18, 1951
Arrival at hospital: 12:15 A.M. Delivered: 4:48 A.M. June 13,
1952

13th August 1952

Dear Mrs.,

I receive a very large number of letters from all sorts and conditions
of people from many corners of the earth, but it is a long time since I
have read a letter with such horrified interest as the one that you have
just written to me.

I can think of nothing more tragic than that a woman who intends to
enjoy this wonderful experience of childbirth should be led into every
possible method of avoiding that enjoyment and making it an unnatural
event. Of course, the gentlemen who attended you and say that 'Read
is O.K., but he goes too far' are those who know nothing whatever
about Read and his work and further probably have no intention whatever of carefully implementing it as he has written it for the comfort
and assistance of women in childbirth.

This we find all over the world and those who know nothing of it are
the greatest critics, and those who know the work are the greatest
supporters and practitioners of it.

The idea of your being given instructions to strain the sphincter
muscles with each successive contraction before the cervix of the uterus
was more than half an inch dilated is the most scandalous misrepresen-
tation of physiological activity that I have ever read; indeed, it is the
one way in which to cause pain and discomfort and the one way in
which to damage the pelvic floor. Strangely enough, it is a very good
method by which a normal labor can be made a slow and extremely
painful performance. If properly conducted and the phenomena of labor understood, a woman might well have her baby in half the time,
without gross discomfort and without any perineal injury.

Another aspect of this is that no woman can possibly put a strain on
an undilated cervix of the uterus without becoming extremely exhausted and if you read carefully in my books the results of exhaustion,
you will see what risks were being taken in advising you in such a manner.

Further, the idea of your being taken to the delivery room to have
your wrists strapped down and your legs strapped up, seems to me to

be a crucifixion of all that is lovely in this most divine accomplishment that is given to human beings. I entirely fail to understand why it should have been painful for you to have been catheterized; we do not consider in the hospital in which I work, that a catheter should give rise to any sensation of discomfort at all to a mother, but rather that the relief of water from the bladder should give her a sense of well-being and satisfaction.

I cannot make any further comments about this case, except that I do wish that you would give me permission without using your name or the place from which you have written, to use this as one of the many examples of the misunderstanding of the physiological processes of labor which give rise to so much trouble not only to mothers and to babies, but in fact sometimes even to the harmony of the family unit.

Happily trouble does not always arise and I do most sincerely hope that you will be one of those who will not suffer in any way from this untidy and undesirable experience.

I would also like you to realize that I am not in any way criticizing your doctors for their performance but rather the manner of their education and the whole trend of outlook towards childbirth that unhappily still exists in some parts of your wonderful country. Men have to carry out the practice that they were educated in, and if they have not time nor inclination to make any further investigations for the benefit and comfort of the women whom they attend, then naturally enough they continue in that teaching which, in my opinion, should have been banished from the medical profession many years ago, and which fortunately is rapidly disappearing where doctors have turned their attention to the relief of women from pain and discomfort.

I only wish you could have seen a woman have her baby this afternoon. I delivered her myself because it was a posterior position and the head would not rotate so it was born with the face to the pubis and weighed just about seven and three quarters pounds. She sat up in bed having had no discomfort that she could speak of; she refused all offers of anesthesia because it was not justified, and when the baby's arms were born she took its hands in hers and even assisted me with the birth of the lower trunk of the baby and its legs by just gently dragging and lifting the baby's arms towards her. Her whole attention was focused upon what to her was the most wonderful thing she had ever seen. The question of discomfort just did not arise. There were no stitches necessary and the loss of blood when the afterbirth was passed was almost negligible, that is to say only four or five ounces at a maximum.

This I might tell you was a woman who was sent to me by her doctor because of her extremely nervous condition, and one who was extremely sensitive also to all forms of painful stimulus. I could not help pulling your letter out of my case and handing it to my assistant to read, and asked him what he thought would happen if such events took place in my practice. His reply was that he thought very probably it would be the death, not to the mother or to the baby but—and there he allowed me to guess to whom he was referring.

All I can do is to offer you my sincere sympathy, but at the same time my congratulations that you have got your baby and that all is well. I wish so much that I could visit _____, Ohio, when next I come to America so that possibly the doctors there as well as many of the mothers might gather together and hear exactly how midwifery is being conducted, not only in my own practice but in the practices of thousands of other medical men and a large number of universities and maternity centres where the truth of physiological processes has been investigated and compared with control cases using other methods.

Your letter has prompted me to write a large letter to you, and I hope you will read it so that my time has not been wasted for I have indeed enjoyed letting off steam when I read of this experience of yours!

My best wishes,

Yours sincerely,
Grantly Dick Read, M.A., M.D., Cantab.

September 8, 1952

Dear Dr. Read,

Do not think me ungrateful for your most welcome answer to my letter. These first twelve weeks of our daughter's life have held such bitterness and despondency for the writer that I hesitate to make any decisions in a moment of irresponsibility.

I think we could have managed if Baby G had not been a 'screamer.' Also, our fair locality set a 50-year heat record during the first 2 1/2 months. What with the above factors and well-meaning relatives, I was eating and sleeping very little.

Dr. Read, please pigeonhole that case history for another month or two until I can gain enough perspective to sit down and write a sequel that makes sense. I'm flattered that you wish to use it, but I would rather you had a knowledge of what followed the birth. Thank you so much for your interest.

Sincerely,

22nd October, 1952

Dear Mrs.,

I will await patiently for a further letter from you. Yours dated the 8th September was, I regret to tell you, no surprise. As I pointed out to you on the 13th August, the treatment that you received is the treatment which causes results of the type from which you are suffering.

Keep your head up and live in reality and you will soon be better.

My best wishes to you,

Yours sincerely,
Grantly Dick Read, M.A., M.D., Cantab.

There was no further correspondence between them.

Correspondence 23

November 16, 1952
Virginia

Dear Dr. Read,

How I wish I could meet you. Several years ago while reading 'The Reader's Digest' I learned of your approach to obstetrics. Immediately I said to myself, 'That makes sense; that's how I'm going to have my children!' That at a time when I hadn't even a husband in sight!!

Now at last my husband and I are eagerly looking forward to April when we're going to welcome the first of *our* next generation. As soon as we thought I was pregnant, we bought your books. Our reaction to these books? How we wish you were here—or we were there! Also we feel that you must be not only a superb obstetrician, but also a wonderful person.

Our greatest problem was getting someone to attend me. My husband, a dentist, is at present with the Navy. We would have had to wait almost two months for a first examination; I didn't want to wait that long, and so we asked about private practitioners. We were referred to a Dr. _____ who turned out to be an obstetrician and gynecologist, something I hadn't wanted, but we had to go on personal recommendation alone. Dr. _____ gave me a very thorough and kindly examination. When we discussed my case, I asked if he would carry me on your method of natural childbirth. His reply was, 'Yes—if you can take it.' That rather stuck in my throat. On reaching home I read the booklet! That was enough for me! I shall send you this under separate cover. You may do whatever you wish with it; I certainly don't want it.

Since knowing that all is in order, and that I'm in good condition for a nice, normal pregnancy, I have changed to Navy care. I did this only after learning that there is at least one obstetrician in the Naval Hospital who recommends your books and your methods. I'll do all in my power to have him attend me.

Why aren't there more doctors who have your sense and understanding? It's very difficult for mothers-to-be who want the joy—and right—of welcoming their babies into the world. Of course there are other mothers (they amaze me). One to whom I was speaking about your way told me, 'I'm not brave enough to do it.' What's brave about it? I'd feel cheated and robbed if I weren't there with a full brass band to welcome this little one of ours! Another mother-to-be (she has one child) to whom I lent our books returned them to me the following day. She told me 'It's too much work—and anyway I don't want to know what's happening to me.' I felt very sorry for her. She it was, too, who told me that her physician doesn't let you rip—he cuts you!!

Enough of my story! I did want to write and thank you, though, for bringing sense and God's intended happiness to childbirth. Not only will today's mothers thank you, but all the countless generations to come. May I give you my heartfelt thanks—I just wish I could shake your hand. Blessings on all your work!

                                                    Sincerely,

31 December 1952

Dear Mrs.,

Your letter which I received quite recently re-introduces me to a constantly recurring problem.

I have no name of any doctor in _____, Virginia, who is known to be an exponent of my methods in fact I know of only one doctor in the state of Virginia and I give his address below, for although you may be a distance away, you could possibly write to him and he might be able to assist you with a name nearer home:

[name and address]

Providing that you are a normal, healthy woman there is no reason at all why you should be unable to have your baby as you wish; 95% of women do and the other 5% are usually the type of person who have very little confidence in anyone and a very uncontrolled emotional state.

No young woman who learns carefully what I have written and who practices deep respiration and relaxation and keeps herself fit by a few physical exercises and a simple balanced diet should have any trouble during pregnancy, and when she comes into labor she must leave the birth of her child to the uterus, patiently alienating herself from its efforts during the first stage to open the birth canal and then assisting it to expel the baby when it calls upon her to give gentle expulsive efforts.

Patience, self-control and ability to work hard if called upon to do is the motto which has guided vast numbers of women to know what a thrilling, magnificent achievement childbirth is.

My best wishes,

                                                    Yours sincerely,
                                    Grantly Dick Read, M.A., M.D., Cantab.

Correspondence 24

Undated - Best Approximation: February or March 1953
Kentucky

Dear Sir,
    With great interest I have read your book 'Childbirth Without Fear'.
I am five months pregnant, and would very much like to have my baby
by your methods. My husband is in the military service, and we live on
an Army post, with a fine hospital and fine doctors, but due to their
workload caused by hundreds of patients in the O.B. Clinic, it seems
impossible to get the supervision and special attention you describe in
your book. I wonder now if it is at all possible to reach the aim of having
a 'Natural Birth', by going entirely by your book, (daily exercises, relaxation, etc.) If it is possible I will, of course, inform my doctor of my
intentions. I would very much appreciate your answer.
                                                          Sincerely yours,

13 April 1953

Dear Mrs.,
    Thank you for your letter which I have just received.
    There are many women who have had their babies quite naturally
with the minimum of discomfort and trouble by reading carefully and
understanding exactly what happens during labor. This enables them
to help themselves without any anticipation of things going wrong.
    The practice of deep breathing and relaxation should be assiduously
carried out and the chapters upon the Phenomena of Labor and the
Conduct of Labor carefully memorized so that the knowledge can be
applied when your baby comes. This will establish a confidence and a
complete absence of fear of this natural function.
    There are many doctors in American Services now who are sympa-
thetic towards assisting their patients to carry out these procedures.
Your difficulty will be, however, to avoid being given drugs in the early
part of labor when even you yourself will realize it is not necessary, for
this is done frequently, and it may not only disturb your concentration
but also your ability to retain the mastership of your own fate. There is

a custom in the U.S.A. to insist upon anaesthetizing a woman for the actual birth of the baby but this should not be done, for the passage of the baby through the outlet of the birth canal does not cause more discomfort than a relaxed woman can bear easily. She will have a sensation of burning and possibly of pressure, but these sensations threaten trouble rather than give it.

I am quite sure if all is normal with you, which of course I am unable to say, you should have your baby as you wish without any trouble, recognizing that I do not preach that it is without discomfort but that such discomfort is so slight that the reward of seeing and hearing your baby born actually outweighs any other thought.

My best wishes,

Yours sincerely,
Grantly Dick Read, M.A., M.D., Cantab.

Correspondence 25

February 15, 1954
Texas

Dear Dr. Read,

I am writing to ask your advice after reading your book, 'Childbirth Without Fear.' I am expecting a baby in July and wish very strongly to have it in the natural way you recommend. I am going to a general practitioner, a personal friend, who is in his 40s (I mention that so you will know he may not be too inflexible in his beliefs), and have told him of my wishes. He has agreed to cooperate with me and says he has delivered a number of babies to women who did not wish anesthetic, but I had the feeling they might have been women who had some personal or religious objection to the anesthetics and just clenched their teeth and bore it, rather than employing the methods of relaxation which you outline.

My question is, is it possible for a woman to be successful in having a baby this way, without undue pain, as long as it is a normal birth, by herself, so to speak, without a doctor completely understanding your methods? I will give you my history as briefly as possible, so that you may judge:

This will be my third baby, I will lack only three months of being 40 when it is born and I am very small, just over 5 feet with a normal weight around 100 pounds. My first baby, which I had at 30, was delivered by the family doctor who delivered me, and except for brief periods of dozing I was conscious until 30 minutes before he was born. I participated consciously in the bearing-down process, but when the doctor arrived 30 minutes before the baby was born, I was frightened by the violence of the contractions and felt I could not get my breath, so I asked him to give me something and was given chloroform. I was conscious enough at the baby's birth to hear them say it was a boy, but that was all.

With the second one, born six years ago, I had a popular obstetrician and went to the hospital around midnight, about three hours before the baby came. He immediately punctured the membranes, which was painful, and gave me a shot, and I knew nothing except for a few brief minutes of groggy consciousness until the next day, nothing at all of the labor room.

In the latter birth, the baby was in a posterior position, and I believe instruments were used to some extent, and in both births there was some laceration, but I don't believe it was extensive. The babies weighed 8 pounds 3 ounces, and 9 pounds three-quarters of an ounce respectively. I am, however, keeping my weight down with this one. After both the other births, I had what I suppose amounted to almost a nervous collapse, as I had little emotional control for sometime afterwards.

One other question I wish to ask is the importance of eliminating red meat from the diet. I did not understand the reason, but could do so if it is important. Normally, we eat beef pretty often, as my husband's business is raising Hereford cattle. If you could find time to answer these questions, however briefly, it would mean a great deal to me, and I am enclosing a stamped, self-addressed envelope for your convenience.

I would like to say that I have the deepest admiration for your courage in crusading for this cause.

23 March 1954

Dear Mrs.,

Thank you very much for your letter of the 15th February which eventually caught up with me.

If you study my book carefully, and particularly the chapter on the 'Conduct of Labor' there is no reason why you should not have your baby as you wish, particularly since your doctor is prepared to let you have your own way.

There are certain points however, which you must keep in mind from beginning to end. Patience in the first stage, relaxing between your contractions, and most important of all, complete self-control throughout. You will find in my book the mention of the emotional menaces, and it is at these time you will find self-control the hardest to maintain by yourself, but you can do it. If you can arrange to have your husband with you as long as possible this will be of the greatest assistance.

I gather from your question on diet that you have not read the new edition of 'Childbirth Without Fear' published by Harpers Bros. in September last year, but if you read this you will see that I have stated in my new chapter on diet that the main thing is to keep to a sensible balanced diet throughout, so please do not worry about eating red meat.

My best wishes to you, good luck, and please let me know the results when the time comes.

Yours sincerely,
Grantly Dick Read, M.A., M.D., Cantab.

Correspondence 26

June 29, 1954
Oregon

Dear Dr. Read—
      Our only child, a son, is 5 1/2.
      I do not become pregnant because I am afraid of childbirth.
      Before I conceived Jeff, I'd read your book. Then I became pregnant and was examined by an obstetrician in Los Angeles. He said my pelvis was shaped narrowly—he pointed it out to the nurse. He told me I might need a cesarean but that he'd let me labor 12 hrs. first.
      Jeff was born 5 hours after I entered the hospital. I entered the hospital about 2 hours after my first pains (for which I took enemas, thinking myself in pain from constipation).
      I think my delivery was fast for a first child.
      But I am terrified of another delivery.
      Jeff's head was very pointed. I heard the Dr say 'forceps' so perhaps he helped Jeff get born.
      When the Doctor said my pelvis was not so good, that's when I felt scared first—that's when the idea of being able to have a delivery like you recommend, dropped away, left me alone and afraid. And I still am alone and afraid about bearing a child. Upbraiding myself as a coward is of course of no value.
      I do want another child. I want the joy of my husband impregnating me; not just having intercourse; I want to nurse an infant again, as I did Jeff—but that darned spinal I had—and not being able to have my husband even in the labor room—what a miserable thing it was to see his face when the nurse told him to kiss me goodbye, that he wouldn't see me again till it was all over—
      Damn it, it's all wrong—humans want to be integrated within themselves and with each other, not all separated—
      I remember the funny scary feeling that part of my brain was disconnected from another part (afterwards).
      Anyway, it was all a nightmare, or I'd've [sic] had another child by now.
      I want you to help me. We haven't money enough at present to enable me to make a long visit—and, I don't know even where you are. I wish you could come by here if you're near here. We're at _____ Boat

Works, where my husband has just started working. It is a good job and the pay is good and we feel quite secure.

I would like to meet you and talk with you, and have you examine me. Then I could figure from there.

One other thing. I would like to adopt a child of 2 or 3 or 4 years, if such an opportunity should ever come about. I tell you this in case you should know of such an opportunity. Even if I were to bear a child a year from now, there would be a great age gap between him and Jeff.

My husband, a very healthy person is 48 years old—thus our chance of finding a youngster via an adoption agency is slight. I am 32.

If we have children of our own again, we'll have two, about two years apart.

I hope you'll write.

Sincerely,

P.S. I am 32 years old.
PPS. Jeff weighed 6 lbs 14 oz at birth

6 July 1954

Dear Mrs.,

I was pleased to get your letter and I feel that I can help you with some fairly strong advice.

If, in five hours, you can have a 6 lb 14 oz baby and that a first one, I am perfectly certain you have got nothing whatever to fear with your second baby, particularly if you follow the principles laid down in my books in relation to diet, exercise and relaxation.

I don't think anyone need be afraid under those circumstances. I assure you the manner of Jeff's birth is quite sufficient to justify your becoming pregnant again within a year much less waiting five and a half years.

I cannot suggest to you whether it would be good advice from me to adopt a baby or not, but all I do know is, and I can tell you right away, that a large number of women who, having been afraid of having another baby for some reason or other which is not clearly understood by them, have adopted babies and within a very short time they are pregnant themselves. It seems they re-awake with tremendous fervor the desire for more children and therefore prepare the body to receive the first possible impregnation.

I like your letter very much and I do hope my advice will be of some help to you. You can't possibly come and see me because I am in England and I don't think I shall be in America until well onwards the end of the year. There is nothing like a good heart and good courage in these matters because the reward is invariably so much greater then you imagine it can be until you have actually brought the thing off.

My best wishes to you and your husband.

Yours sincerely,
Grantly Dick Read, M.A., M.D., Cantab.

Correspondence 27

3 August 1955
Liverpool

Dear Dr. Read,

I hope you will excuse me writing to you but I am a devoted follower of your teachings on natural childbirth. I have a son of 4 1/2 who was born naturally when I was 22 but since then I have had 3 abortions at between 7 and 9 weeks. I had treatment from the fourth week in the last 2 cases. . . . On the last occasion I was admitted to the hospital and had a D&C operation.

I am now 12 weeks pregnant and have just had two weeks in bed as a precautionary measure. Opinion seems to be divided between my having a retroversion or a 'very hostile womb.'

I have been reading your book again and would very much appreciate your advice as to the advisability of starting the exercises and relaxation. You mention an early start with relaxation to be beneficial in helping nervous symptoms (and I have acute nausea and occasional retching without food), but say 'unless there is no retroversion.'

I apologise for troubling you but am very anxious to make this a successful pregnancy and my own doctor is a very busy G.P. with no time for what he would call 'fancy notions.' I know it is not medical etiquette for a doctor to recommend another, but if you know anyone or any establishment which follows your teaching, in this area, I should be most grateful of the information.

Yours most sincerely,

6 August 1955

Dear Mrs.,

Thank you for your letter. It does sound very much to me as if there is a considerable if not obvious emotional influence in your having had three abortions between seven and nine weeks.

Therefore I should advise you most strongly to practice relaxation quietly and to realize that there is no reason at all why you should abort. I take it that you live a pretty healthy life, and avoid, as far as possible for the present time, intercourse with your husband and also excessive alcohol. I don't think I should concentrate your thoughts too much on

CMAC:PP/GDR/D.44

the pregnancy but let it come on as it will, and particularly about the time when your periods would probably be due, go to bed even if you have to stay there for a week.

That is the usual treatment of this, and I don't think I am offending any doctor because I am no longer a practising doctor myself, and I hope that will have some influence.

I enclose the name of a doctor who has been recommended to me as being a follower of this teaching [near where you live].

Yours sincerely

Grantly Dick Read, M.A., M.D., Cantab.

14 August 1955

Dear Dr. Read,

Thank you so much for your most helpful letter. I have been practising relaxing each afternoon and have lost all my sickness and apprehension about aborting.

I am following the diet you advise in your book and thought I would start the exercises after the 16th week which I have managed to spend in bed.

Your book is referred to constantly in this house and I only hope you are preparing some other work for publication; I feel your views on the lying-in period and post-natal exercises and advice on breast feeding would be eagerly followed by the thousands of women who conduct their pregnancy and labour on the knowledge gained from your books.

Your letter has given me faith that I can carry this child, and I shall do all I can to repay you by advocating natural childbirth to my friends even more strongly than I have in the past.

Yours sincerely,

22 August 1955

Dear Mrs.,

Dr. Dick Read received your letter as he was leaving for a lecture tour, and he has asked me to write to you saying how pleased he is that you have gained confidence in yourself and are feeling so much better.

You ask about any other works in preparation and at the present time there is a small handbook with the publisher which should be out in the near future entitled 'Antenatal Illustrated' which title is self-explanatory. I don't know whether you have the third edition of 'Childbirth Without Fear' published in August 1954, but if you have not, you would be able to find in that later edition a chapter devoted to breast-feeding which would be of interest to you, as well as notes on post-natal care. Dr. Dick Read completely revised 'Childbirth Without Fear' for this third edition so you would find a lot of new material in it.

Dr. Dick Read does hope that in the fullness of time you will write and let him know how everything goes on with you.

Yours sincerely,
Secretary to Grantly Dick Read

11 April 1956

Dear Dr. Dick Read,

I am glad to write to tell you that I was delivered of an 8 lb daughter two months ago. I followed all your advice re exercises and diet, and although I didn't feel to fit while I was pregnant, my labour was short and I was perfectly alright after she was born. In fact, the midwife said it was a waste of time coming as my pulse or temperature never varied even though my son had bronchitis, suspected appendicitis, and a touch of enteritis in the two weeks following the birth.

The baby is doing well. She is very contented and gained 10 oz last week. I know I should not have been able to bring her naturally if it had not been for the confidence I gained from reading and rereading your books, and I'm sure successful breast feeding depends to a large extent on the feeling of 'one-ness' with your child which results from a natural birth.

Many thanks again for all your help.

Yours sincerely,

16 April 1956

Dear Mrs.,

Thank you very much for your letter of April 11, and I am so glad to see that you had a successful pregnancy although not feeling too fit, and that you achieved your desire of a second natural birth.

I am so glad to see that you are breast feeding your little daughter, and I do hope that you will have no further troubles with your own health.

Do write and let me know if and when you have any further additions to what I am sure is a very happy family life.

My best wishes to you and your husband, to say nothing of your children.

Yours sincerely,
Grantly Dick Read, M.A., M.D., Cantab.

Section 5

Disagreeing with the Dick-Read Method

"Maybe it 'wasn't meant to hurt' but it does. It hurts like the devil!"

*W*hen women read Dick-Read's books and prepared themselves for a natural childbirth, they believed that they would be part of the 95%-97% of women who would achieve childbirth without drugs. However, once labor started, some found they were in pain and needed more than breathing exercises and relaxation techniques for assistance. Women wrote of feeling cheated and tricked by his writings. Others wrote of the sheer disappointment they felt in themselves. He even received correspondence suggesting themes and improvements for future editions of his books. Dick-Read's responses included sympathy for their having to take the drugs, suggestions that they were not properly prepared for the hard work of natural childbirth, and took the opportunity to promote his antenatal literature.

Correspondence 28

March 28, 1947
New York

Dear Dr. Read,

I have just finished reading 'Childbirth Without Fear' and am very impressed. However, being seven months pregnant with a second child I feel there was much in the book not only not addressed to me, but that I would have preferred to remain ignorant of. I) The danger of many drugs (I do not know how I was 'doped' last time but now have the seed of a new fear of what will be used this time. Yet without your theory in practice fear to do without it.) 2) The 'abnormality' of forceps—(which I had last time to no apparent harm to my baby or me—but now makes me wonder—) 3) Many of the extreme horrors of 'natural' childbirth of which I had been happily unaware. 4) Why don't you write a book exclusively for the pregnant and lay reader keeping in mind the cultural predisposition's of her obstetrician and aiming not to have her lose faith in him as your present book does—keep in mind too—that she will probably not get the sympathetic bedside care which you give. I still think you could inspire the fearless approach and perhaps suggest tactful ways that the patient could request of the nurse or doctor in attendance to give your kind of helpful hints (I'm sure very few doctors would be pleased to hear—'If Dr. Read were here he would do thus and so. . . .')

There is a crying need for a good book dealing with pre-natal emotional preparation for pregnancy itself and motherhood as well as labor for the lay reader. I am convinced you are the person to write it.

Very truly yours,

P.S. The English title 'Revelation in Childbirth' reflects the positive contribution of your book far better than its American title.

29th April 1947

Dear Mrs.,

Your letter dated one month ago today has just arrived. It is so refreshing to receive a letter which is not full of enthusiasm and enthusiasm only that I propose to answer it at length, and expressing at the same time my gratitude for your comments. I do not disagree with a single word that you write and am fully aware of the quandary in which certain parts of the book called 'Childbirth Without Fear' must place you under the circumstances. When I was in New York in January and February of this year this aspect of that particular book was freely discussed with Miss Hazel Corbin and Miss Stevens who are at the New York Maternity Center, 654 Madison Avenue. These two extremely capable and experienced women saw at once that many American women might be disturbed by some of my arguments. It is undoubtedly true for there is much more interference in normal labor in America than in this country.

We aim primarily at the natural and normal in as much as our first object is to prevent a mother suffering. To that end we employ means which are least likely to necessitate interference and thereby, in a certain number of cases, injury to both mother and child or one or the other. My teaching enables that to be done in a large majority of normal cases. If there is any obstetric abnormality which may occur in three to five percent only, then my teaching does not apply.

I have a small book coming out next month in England which so far as possible will eliminate the story of the difficult and abnormal labors and lay stress on the means by which simplicity can be attained. I am just writing a book exactly upon the lines which you demand and I hope it will be successful in eliminating the fear and a good deal of the misunderstanding of childbirth.

Now I must [agree] with you how this thing has come about in 'Childbirth Without Fear.' I agree with you too that I prefer the name of the English edition to that which my American publishers chose for themselves. I am sure you will recognize that having been at this particular work for just on thirty years, I have met with all the opposition and prejudice that a pioneer of a new line of thought is subjected to. It was not enough for me just to state my case. My arguments and to be clearly expounded and in order to do that I could not leave out those [important] results which experience had shown to occur in the practice of obstetrics with an approach that diametrically differed from mine. That book was not really written primarily for the lay public but for the medical profession and those who deal with childbearing women. I was very astonished myself when after a relatively short time thousands of copies were found to be selling to the lay public all over the world. Those who are critical rarely write; those who are grateful and enthusiastic write in large numbers and I receive hundreds of letters from all the English speaking races of gratitude for the applications of this approach to midwifery—perhaps that is why I value your letter much more than most of them.

I am grieved, however, if as you obviously have with a clear sight both into the pros and the cons of the case, that you have suffered any emotional turmoil from what I have written. There are many doctors in America now who are practicing obstetrics with my approach and who are sending me excellent reports of results attained but, as you are fully aware, a large percentage still believe in the mechanization of a natural process; that brings us rather in touch with the philosophical aspect of childbirth and all it means. Please do not feel that I infer that every woman whose child is delivered with forceps operation and who is unconscious or without feeling at the time, must suffer any harm or her child, but statistically it has been shown that the percentage of those who do suffer harm is too high to justify this as an invariable approach when there is another and simpler method by which the law of nature can be observed without either distress or injury to the mother or the child.

Your baby should not have arrived by the time that you receive this letter and I would be grateful if you could find opportunity for calling upon Miss Hazel Corbin and Miss Stevens at the Maternity Center Association and discussing this matter with them. They are doing very great work for obstetrics in America and I think that you would not feel one moment of your time with them was wasted. If without presumption I may make one short suggestion to you; study carefully the chapter in 'Childbirth Without Fear' on the Conduct of Labour, realize the stages and the progress of childbirth and then exercise during the first stage patience and allow your uterus to prepare itself to be opened; self control so that the sensations which you desire to push your baby freely into the world knowing that there is not necessity for pain if you allow the natural machine of childbearing to work undisturbed by any emotional excess that you may give rise to in your mind.

My best wishes to you and again thank you for your commentary.

Yours sincerely,
Grantly Dick Read, M.A., M.D., Cantab.

September 16, 1947

Dear Dr. Dick Read,

I have waited until my baby arrived to acknowledge your very kind letter of April 29th. I found it charming indeed and conscientious of you to write when I received it; now it has made *you* my obstetrician for indeed, armed with your letter, your book, pamphlets of your speeches in N.Y. which Miss Stevens gave me, even in the delivery room, you were indeed there in spirit.

May I tell you about it in detail. I would like you to know how well your idea works even against every [handicap].

After receiving your letter, I spoke to Miss Stevens at length—she was very kind and encouraging. I discussed your book with my obstetrician who is the head of Gynecology at one of N.Y.C. biggest hospitals. He thought your idea an interesting one, but was convinced it wouldn't work. Frankly, I was rather skeptical myself—but I wanted to try it—though I had done none of the exercises and was worried about the unsympathetic attitude of the doctor.

During that long first stage of labor (nearly 20 hours) I reread your letter repeatedly, reread your chapters on Conduct of Labor and Relaxation and gave the pamphlets to attending nurses—I was proselytizing the whole time. Fortunately, there was one sympathetic nurse in attendance fairly early in the labor and I got into the 'habit' of relaxing on the contractions. While she was there, there was a woman in the adjoining labor room who was screaming painfully—I thought—Heavens I'm doing so well only because this is the beginning—my intense ones haven't started yet. I got panicky—tensed up and the next contraction was a labor pain. I think out of self-preservation as much as compassion for my suffering neighbor I asked the nurse to go to her for a few minutes, tell her about your idea, calm her down, tell her to relax and tell her it is working with me. The nurse spent ten minutes with her and the woman did not deliver until several hours later, I didn't even hear her groan, though before that her yells had been bloodcurdling. I was thrilled—in the midst of labor I had 'spread the gospel' to a person who had never heard of you or your ideas and helped her with such brief and indirect tutelage—'A learning mind makes the best teacher.'

Unfortunately, that one nice nurse went off duty seven hours before my baby was born, and my efforts at converting nurses was discouraging. I had to *fight* with them not to give me an analgesic, I was left alone hours on end and then my longing for a kind word or moral support came from your letter—I read it or thought about it after every frustration like the time a nurse was passing as a contraction was starting and I asked her to please hold my hand for a minute (I had found that a big help while the sympathetic nurse was there)—and she said casually 'I'm best to hold on to the bed post.' Nevertheless with the exception of that one real pain when that other woman was vocalizing her distress, I had nothing but intense 'contractions' similar to a stiff 'muscle bound' after too much exercise. And some people were impressed! And the resident doctor had heard your lectures and was very interested how well it was working.

At this point may I tell you how mistaken you were in a point in your book. I winced when I read the passage where you stated in labor you can tell the real fibber [sic] of a woman "The 'I can't and I won't' and the 'I can and I will' types." For during my labor with my first child I was definitely the former where this time I was distinctly the second. Even that depends on a woman's approach and state of mind!

I was having second stage contractions and rather enjoying my sense of accomplishment when my doctor arrived. He is a nice person and is considered a very fine doctor but he is one these 'big shots' who rush in for delivery, always with deep anesthesia, episiotomy and forceps. He was unimpressed when I told him I was enjoying this labor and that I couldn't believe the baby was ready for delivery. When he said 'close enough' I reminded him politely that I wanted a natural birth.

When the ether mask was forced on my face I got furious. The nurse told me several days later that I was thoroughly insulting to the doctor—told him to go back to his damn office. (I had noticed on the clock that I was interrupting his office hours) and that all I needed for this delivery was a policeman to cut the cord. It was exactly what I had feared when I wrote to you after first reading your book. I had lost confidence in my doctor—I was quoting you frantically and had thoroughly annoyed him. Knowing this, my fury was mixed with guilty feelings when I first saw my baby the next day. The little fellow's head was a mass of black and blue forceps marks and there was a cut on his forehead. I felt that I had angered the doctor so that he was unconsciously, unduly rough. Whereas, the first time I saw my first child, I was thrilled and happy—something akin to the ecstasy you describe but not as intense as when it immediately follows the concentration of labor—this time my exhilaration turned to fury when I realized how cruelly unnecessary were all those bruises the black eye and the cut.

My labor was wonderful, my delivery awful (mentally not physically—I was 'out') and I felt cheated.

I hope to have another baby in about two years and this time with the help of Miss Stevens I am going to shop until I find a disciple of yours. I talk 'Dick Read' to every pregnant girl I meet—but even when I've convinced them, what good is it if their doctor won't co-operate. The best is that their labor will be easier.

At least now I fully appreciate the crusading you evinced in your book and I objected to before! I am most interested in the new book which you mentioned and would very much appreciate knowing the title and publisher for despite the fact that you said you appreciated my first letter precisely for its critical tone, I must now confess that I am an unconditional 'fan' of yours.

I do hope your new book contains as much on the state of mind throughout the entire pregnancy as on the labor itself. I have found that women who feel well for the nine months have far easier labors than those who have been ill. And yet, just as one 'expects' labor to be painful, most women wait for nausea as a sign of pregnancy and there is nothing so likely to induce it as expecting it. Every book I have read on prenatal care has had suggestions for treating discomforts, never one suggesting that a woman is reaching a fulfillment during pregnancy and should feel better than ever. Another sad commentary in this country is the small percentage of mothers who breast feed their children. Most of the American obstetricians are against it and although the pediatricians are in favor of nursing by the time the pediatrician is called in the new mother has been oriented toward the bottle.

May I make a suggestion where I disagree with your prenatal approach. You mentioned several times in your chapters 'Records of Cases' that a mother was so delighted the baby was the sex she had hoped for. After all there is only a 50% chance of winning on that score, isn't it foolish to 'root' for a boy or girl. It is just as easy to be convinced it doesn't matter what sex the child is and thereby eliminate disappointments which may have far reaching psychological effects on the new members of the family. A far more healthy subject for speculation is the potential personality of the baby, girl or boy, will it be gentle and placid, active and sensitive, etc. etc. It prepares the parents better for taking the new child for what he or she is and makes for a more sensitive handling of personality differences. And throughout life, the personality of the child will affect the parents far more than the matter of purchasing either dresses or trousers.

Dr. Dick Read, the charm and wisdom of your personality are so evident in your writing. I do hope your new book will serve as a personal letter to very many pregnant women. I hope that thereby you will become their obstetrician in spirit as you were mine and that soon your book will be considered compulsory reading for every mother-to-be.

Most sincerely,

28th September 1947

Dear Mrs.,

I was most grateful for your letter. I consider it to be a classical example of a large number I have received from the United States. Happily a few doctors have been willing to believe and understand. Today in the same mail as yours I received a letter from Boston, Mass., Dr. _____, of the Harvard Unit, who is expert in the use of my procedures, saw a patient of mine who is going to have a baby. Being on the Boston Lying-In Hospital Staff, he is unable to do private work. He therefore sent her to Dr. _____. Dr. _____ I am glad to say is a broad-minded man, for I read 'although he does not practice your methods exclusively he does his best to emulate them when requested.' Also by the same post I had a communication from Dr. _____, of the Grace New Haven Community Hospital, where the Yale Medical Units work. He writes that although they have not had opportunity for continuing a large number of physiological labors 'I am already utterly convinced that the use of your techniques throughout pregnancy and labor is of inestimable value.'

In this time, the women of America will not be subjected to the misunderstandings of our profession. During last night two of my patients had their first babies without a thought of anesthetic, without a murmur of intolerance of any sensation they experienced. They held their children's hands before it was possible to tell whether they were daughters or sons. I was at a third case whilst my Assistant looked after the two I have mentioned; the personality factor was therefore ruled out. It was the simple happiness of physiological events carried out by two young women who knew what to do, who understood what was going on and who were assisted to interpret all their sensations in the light of truth.

Last week Colonel _____ of the American Medical Mission, came to the Hospital where I work and discussed with my patients their experiences during labor. One and all were ready for another baby as soon as possible, and the question of pain, laceration or exhaustion was in each case met with a smile of incredulity that such things should still happen as a routine in a civilized country. Colonel _____ told me before he left that nothing in the world could have made him believe this miracle (as he described it) unless he had seen and talked to the patients and seen their babies in some cases a few hours after the births have taken place.

So you need have no fear that what you are believing and preaching has anything of a flaw or a fallacy about it. May I say with all respect and a real admiration for your courage in the most difficult circumstances, that you have touched the fringe of the real beauty of childbirth. I am sure you will understand me better than most women when I repeat to you what so many women say to me after the arrival of their child—'It was more a spiritual experience to me than a physical ordeal.' Mere man can only wonder and perhaps, if familiar with these things, envy the noble souls whose patience, self-control and fortitude have enabled them to reap the just reward of exercising the highest qualities of womanhood.

I send you my most cordial regards, and wish so much that thousands of the women of your great country could know of your experiences, your thoughts and your beliefs, for it is upon such things that not only the future of families will depend, but also the structure and philosophy of the greatest peoples of the world.

Yours very sincerely,

Grantly Dick Read, M.A., M.D., Cantab.

Correspondence 29

June 2, 1947
Maryland

Dear Dr. Read,

During my last month of pregnancy I read the condensation of your book 'Childbirth Without Fear' with great interest. It expounded a theory I had long held with—now, in a short time, I was going to prove it to myself. My friends who are already mothers didn't try to dissuade me—they said that they'd pay head when I came home from the hospital and reiterated.

I arrived at the hospital in a high state of expectancy, happy in the thought that soon my daughter would be nuzzling at my breast. To while [sic] away the time in the labor room I read a book, and tried to convince the woman in the other bed that there was nothing to fear. She was having a rather rough time of it. But that didn't shake my faith one iota. The nurses on the floor didn't abate it either (O.B. laboring women.) Their 'there's nothing to it' was in accord with my own thinking.

When my slight discomfort began to be more disturbing, I started applying the 'relax' theory. The harder the pains, the more I tried to relax. I'd always prided myself on the ability to relax completely. After ten hours I realized that it was no good, and at the end of eighteen hours, when the baby was finally born, I had a turnabout in my thinking. When I had started I was planning to ask them not to use an anesthetic, but at the end, I was begging for it. And mine was considered an 'easy' birth.

Now I know, of course, that some people don't feel pain as others do—and more power to them. But for my money the theory of 'relax and enjoy it' doesn't hold water. I tried and I know. And one who has never been a mother, no matter how much observation, can never appreciate what it is like.

Maybe it 'wasn't meant to hurt' but it *does*. It hurts like the devil!

Sincerely,

No Response

CMAC:PP/GDR/D.106

Correspondence 30

20 October 1949
East Yorks

Dear Dr. Read,

I am writing to thank you for the help I received by reading your book on natural childbirth. I had my first little girl in 1947 and was very disappointed when I was given anesthetic and I had no experience of the actual birth. It seemed very un-natural to me and when I read your book last year I was very pleased that you agreed that if possible birth should be natural and determined to have my second baby that way. I mentioned this to my doctor and he said that in his opinion only one woman in a hundred could do it, but I was determined to carry on. My midwife was in favor of it however. My labor pains started about 10:15 pm [on] September 3. They came regularly every 10 minutes, and for the first hour I relaxed on the couch and listened to a radio play, then they speeded up to every 5 minutes, so I relaxed on the bed and at 11:40 pm my husband rang for the midwife. I slept a bit during the first stage which was most helpful as I felt rather tired. The midwife allowed me to go to the bathroom to pass water and I think the head crowned then for it was a very unpleasant feeling, and I'm afraid I cried a bit and thought I should not be able to manage. Real pains started in earnest now and I started to call out, but nurse showed me how to bear down on them and not waste them. After this it was a tough struggle, my waters broke and I worked really hard—so did nurse. In between the contractions I still managed to relax a little and gather up strength for the next effort. I experienced the feeling that I should burst but having read about it in your book I was not alarmed and knew the birth was near. Baby G arrived at 2:45 am and it was most exciting to feel when she actually arrived, and her first splutter and cry was very wonderful. Soon she was wrapped in a blanket and snuggled in my arms and I was wonderfully happy. The fight was tough going and I felt battered at the time and it did hurt but a different sort of pain more like bruising and after the birth I soon forgot them. The only part of your plan I could not accept was that I should see my baby before she was wrapped up. I didn't want to until she was bathed apart from that I am heartily in agreement with you, and I am very glad to have had your help. My friends find it difficult to believe that I did not even use gas and air relief and I am recommending your book to them, and if I have another baby I hope that I shall have her as happily as this one. If any of my experience is helpful to your practice please pass it on to them as I would like to feel I am helping your campaign.

Yours sincerely,

11 January 1950

Dear Mrs.,

It is very kind of you to have written to me at such length about the birth of your baby. It always gives me pleasure to read from mothers that I have not known that they have derived some benefit from following the teaching.

We have the statistics from all over the world showing that 90% of women are able to comply physiologically if properly cared for and prepared.

I am sure you will never forget your experience and you will be interested to see the difference in the natures of your two children. Look a placid and healthy baby in Baby G and also take notice of your husband's attitude towards her.

My best wishes to you and once more my congratulations that you have dared to persevere in what you have known to be right.

Yours sincerely,
Grantly Dick Read, M.A., M.D., Cantab.

Correspondence 31

November 1, 1949
New Jersey

Dear Doctor Read,

You have probably had many comments both pro and con on your book 'Childbirth Without Fear', but I hope this latest one does not find its way into your wastebasket without being read, as, although I am inclined to disagree with your premise that childbirth is natural, pain-less both from experience and natural observation I should like to have you know that you have given much food for thought in throwing into the forum for discussion and alteration the stoneage treatment of twen-tieth century maternity patients. Also, until I have seen your ideas in operation, out of deference and respect for your obvious humanity, (as well as common sense - you may be right and I may be wrong) I will not allow myself an absolute opinion but one 'subject to change without notice' like a Sunday train.

I believe that childbirth *should* be painless only it isn't. The easiest pregnancy and childbirth is not easy or pleasant. No matter how much you pretend to yourself that you enjoy every meal, the fact is, you don't. You feel like a gastric ulcer patient even though you tell yourself it is worth it: see what you will get in a few months and your digestion, too? You are heavy and clumsy—that cannot be avoided—and you seem to lose control of your feet. Your features coarsen and you look a sight, while the chances are that if your circumstances are moderate and you cannot afford the right diet or maternity garments, that is how you are going to look all your life. (Not that you would mind so much if your husband lost his figure and health when you lost yours; it seems almost too much to look and feel as you do when pregnant and then listen to men brag about their virility and the proper place for women in the scheme of life.)

It is mainly the attitude of the human male which brings about that 'absurd humility' you speak of. You have only to sit in a club room, hotel lobby or public conveyance and listen to the comments of the throng to understand one of the reasons why pregnant women dislike being seen. A second reason is that a pregnant woman is an unforgettable offense to herself. She smells, a penetrating 'baby' odor of which she is always

CMAC:PP/GDR/D.99

conscious. It clings to body, clothes and bed despite any amount of airing, bathing and changing. Thirdly, it is probably a partial holdover from dawn man days to crawl into a cave and hide during a period when vulnerable to attack. All female animals do it, even the domesticated ones if they are given the opportunity. (How many times are farm children sent to find the cow which has hidden herself to bear her calf in secret safety?)

If the baby is healthy its kicking batters one into complete exhaustion, yet it cannot be put into another room and left until the prospective mother is rested enough to pick up her burden and carry on. I have kicked my husband awake out of pure hatred and jealously during sleepless hours of pregnancy because he could and I couldn't.

My husband was very patient with me during my pregnancies—when he was home. He was a few thousand miles away when each of the first two were born, and just as well probably, because I would certainly have spoiled our married life by telling him exactly what I thought about men, sex, birth and life. A sensitive person of either sex does not like to feel that they are regarded only as a breeding animal, and stripping aside such sentiments as the beauty of motherhood, the nation's need, the future of the race, my husband's attitude and yours breaks down to the statement that 'breeding is the one and only duty of woman.' True or false, the idea of being a baby factory in an age when the child no longer belongs to the mother - if it ever has - but is in reality the property of the state, is one of exceeding revulsion. Would you like to spend all your time fathering children who would never belong to you, and give up your work, which I am sure you love, simply because nature gave you the means to reproduce yourself? Women are people, too, and as much entitled to careers apart from the biological function nature has assigned to them as men. Nor would you, nor any man above the level of an animal, like the mindless creature who thought only of reproducing herself in an erotic frenzy without regard to circumstances.

As for throwing discretion to the winds, it has been done by selfish men throughout history, but never in the history of man has there been a time when one could bring a child into the world without discretion. There probably never will be, although I hope for it. . . .

Both my husband and I spring from sane, healthy, long-lived families of above average mentality and - apparently - fertility: we run to large families. My husband is a country man with a country man's confidence and unconcern about birth, a perfectly natural process occurring daily, a temporary condition ending with great rewards, a condition as far as he knows happily endure[d] by his mother who had nine children. . . .

As far as I can see, children are all work, much expense, worry, and frequent sorrow, even if they all grow up, turn out well, keep their health, and marry wisely.

As my mother had so many children [8], I was naturally brought up to believe that children were normal and inevitable, that women without children were crippled, selfish, or idle, while those who complained about pain were simply lazy excuse makers. Then I had three children.

As far as I know, all three births were quite usual, though with slightly longer labors than most. In the first two, my self control was excellent, in the last case I had none. In all cases, part of my mind was observing with complete detachment, all my sensations, emotions, reactions, and environment, and adding them up not—to me—reasonable conclusions. I was able to in every case to subtract effort from pain or vice versa and came to the conclusion that Nature never intended birth to be easy except for her favorites. . . .

Nor do I believe that primitive women had painless childbirth. They endured grimly, dumbly, like other animals and those who didn't, or couldn't, or wouldn't just died. They endured what they could not mend, or interpret, or feared to express because of greater fears of wild animals, brutal mates and death.

A woman with childbirth behind her is willing to concede that 'it is not so bad' or even allow herself to believe that she had no pangs. I have lied that way to comfort my husband, my family, and my doctor, as the poor dears congratulated me on having come through so comfortably.

Both my second and third child were conceived against my will, *as most children are,* although many women will not admit it because they hate to 'lose face' among their associates by a further admission that their husbands forced their submission. It *is* a shameful thing to admit that your husband has no consideration for your wishes, or no control over his appetites. But it is still worse not to realize that such behavior is due to ignorance, lack of training and a complete, natural, inability to understand a woman's point of view because they are not women. Before any condition can be changed or altered, the basic natural facts must be taken into consideration.

To continue: according to your teachings, I had every reason to believe that my second birth would be difficult and unhappy. I was greatly frightened because my baby started on its way ahead of time. I could not get in touch with the doctor I had chosen, and, in whom I had learned confidence, but was obliged to obtain the services of another whom I did not know and of whom I was afraid. They left me alone in the room, and I was in dread lest the baby arrive and I could not get help; also I was afraid the baby might die because it was premature. Yet in spite of all these things, the labor was not hard, the 'hard' labor did not pain at all, and the baby was halfway into the world before I reached the delivery room. I asked them not to administer anesthetic until I asked for it, and it was not until my baby was springing into the world that they dimmed my perception. Within minutes of her birth I was feeling and handling her.

I can discern no noticeable difference in my emotional attitude towards this child, whom I held in my hands at birth and those which I did not. No doubt I appeared to be in a state of wild delight when I saw all three of them, but believe me, Doctor, my delight, to be quite honest, in seeing them, was mainly composed of exquisite relief that they were out in the world and not a burden within me. . . . As for really loving the babe for itself, ask any woman at what age she liked her baby best and you will discover when she became attached to it without the compulsion of precedent which rules that a mother *must* love her child the moment it is born or she is an unnatural creature.

I will not shock you by telling you at which age I like my children best.

Nor can I agree that the manner of birth has much to do with the infant's disposition as long as it is born whole. Despite two difficult births and one 'easy', all three of my babies were angelical, no trouble at all. Most babies I have seen are like that. . . .

I notice that you assume a sex drive in women, by the way, quite incompatible with nature and the responsibility of the female parent towards her young.

Almost any woman can have a baby all by herself, endure it, and live through it. In fact, the knowledge that she is on her own, probably gives her desperation the same adrenal lift which lends wings to the feet of fleeing terror. But because a woman can struggle through is no excuse for minimizing her pains, which do exist, I assure you, or for inferring that she is a coward if she will not put up with and make the best of it; or for condemning the whole of womankind as hypochondriacs because of the difference in the intensity of pain each can endure.

The mating itself must make a difference in the ease of the birth as humans are not of regulation size. There is enough difference between them, apart from variations due to diet and environment to make all the difference between pain and hellish effort according to the size, shape and skeletal peculiarities of both parents. . . .

However, if I have another baby, I shall certainly try your methods from intellectual curiosity. Indeed, I am almost tempted to have another baby simply as an experiment, using your theory but not your point of view. You believe the race has retrogressed, rather than progressed. I am more optimistic. I believe that the mental therapy you suggest is one which only a highly civilized race could use and I am sure that now that we have streamlined our artifacts, we will streamline ourselves to match. Intelligent women, perhaps using your book as a guidebook towards it, will learn a mental control of their functions which will enable them to minimize pain or even block it off by closing their minds against it. That 'tearing' sensation which you insist is not a pain is no joke. I have split the webbing between my fingers at times, but find the comparison very poor. The relief from the 'tearing' makes one ready to weep for joy that it is over but does not make it easier, more bearable, less *painful*. However, when you know that the worst is about over, most women will take the pain to ether, as long as they can stand it, or are not too worn down from the labor, but the fact that a woman refused ether, claims she has no pain, may mean nothing but excellent endurance. The pain a woman can stand without complaint, no matter how it hurts, she calls 'no pain'. (Ask about it.)

Perhaps operations of all kinds will be performed someday by methods similar to yours without the use of anesthesia. It is true, your idea is not exactly new, but it is the first practical application of, shall I say, acrobatic yoga?

It is a pity that your methods must always be a theory, personally, no matter how practically applied otherwise the fact that you cannot make a physical demonstration upon yourself in this instance must give you either an unreasonable confidence or a niggling doubt. . . .

I hope you will forgive the poor spelling and typing, as well as the general layout of this letter. With three small children it is difficult even to write a note, let alone a letter of such length, especially as our latest baby is only just over four months and a large, heavy child. Caring for him is very tiring. He is over twenty six inches long and weighs twenty pounds, and is such a handsome, progressive good natured infant that we cannot help being very proud of him.

Good luck, Doctor Read, I sincerely hope you are right for my daughter's sake, for, as it is, every woman regrets her daughters because of the ordeal which lies ahead of them. An ordeal which may be made much worse by circumstance, for not all men are kind, nor financially sound and disease is no respecter of persons of any degree.

Very truly yours,

29 December 1949

Dear Mrs.,

Your letter did not find my waste paper basket. It is very interesting and represents one of a considerable number I have received from women during the last thirty years.

My first suggestion to you is have another baby and go and see Dr.
_____, and if possible, arrange for him or someone who is equally pro-
ficient in the art, to assist you to carry out the procedures I lay down.

I am more than willing to accept that everything you write concerning childbirth is applicable to Mrs. [her name], in childbirth. I entirely
disagree with you in much that you say and I am a little surprised to find
in a letter of such intelligence your suggestion 'It is a pity I cannot have
a baby myself.' This remark has been made in correspondence in second class daily papers for at least twenty years. My observations are
not my own. They are the sum of comments and letters of thousands
of women of all nationalities. They also represent all classes, from gyp-
sies to duchesses.

Most of my important observations have been corroborated by medical women, a large number of who have been under my care at the
birth of their children. I regret too that I am unable to be a mother, but
I do not suggest that the fact implies any weakness in a thesis which
has brought happiness and confidence and relief of pain in variable measure to such a vast number of women.

Your attitude towards the appearance of a woman in pregnancy only
demonstrates one fact and that is that you have had little or no experience of those who are properly prepared and guided through pregnancy
and that your own experience was unfortunate.

Possibly one of the greatest assets of the ante natal care of a woman
is that she is justified in the pride that she has of her appearance during
pregnancy. She is taught correct posture, she is given those exercises
which do not allow her shape to become ungainly, and many other things
that I need not outline. If you have been sufficiently unfortunate to
come into contact and hear the comments of men who are rather cyni-
cal or adversely critical of pregnant women I suggest that you should
judge the men and not pregnancy.

I do not for one moment disagree with you that anyone whose attitude towards childbirth and whose beliefs and whose introspective
conceptions of what childbirth is or is intended to be, is likely to have
her baby without very considerable physical and emotional discomfort.
As you rightly say, Nature may prescribe painful childbirth and even
death to those unworthy to survive. Nature may also prescribe painful
childbirth as a reward of misunderstanding of its designs.

It appears from your letter that you have not been cared for by medical
men who understand the processes of physiological childbirth. You have
been neither prepared nor assisted in the manner which is laid down in
the book that you have read. . . .

Because you have not been able to appreciate all the natural emotional phenomena that come within the design of Nature in relation to this concept of childbirth, I hope you will not presume or assume that you are a fair example of the motherhood of today. If it is your wish to assist your daughters to undertake, when their time comes, motherhood with a sense of ambition and enjoyment, I feel that you will have to see it through different spectacles before they are given the best possible education to that end. They may agree with you that a woman is not [for breeding] only but a human being, demanding a career in this life. My point of view is that a woman who is blessed with the ability to marry for love of the man whom she hopes to be the father of her children and in due course to have these children, that they in due course may live unselfish and purposeful and, therefore, successful lives. It is such people who are the foundations of society and who by creating well knit family units establish a philosophy in the environment in which they live which makes for happiness and mental health.

Thank you very much for writing to me. So many letters that I receive are simply of adulation. To have the criticisms of one who is not in the ordinary run is most refreshing.

Yours sincerely,
Grantly Dick Read, M.A., M.D., Cantab.

Correspondence 32

Undated [Best approximation is in the 1950s]
Newtown

Dear Doctor Read:

All this talk about woman [sic] having a happy time when they bring
a child into the world is a lot of *bull* unless of course we could all have
Dr. Read in attendance. Bringing my first child into the world was the
most painful and horrible experience I ever had. I had a beautiful baby
boy nine pounds eight. This experience left me quite miserable. But like
the pilot who is sent up again after the crash I had a very strong desire
to have another baby. So my husband and I arranged it. I was very
happy. From the beginning of this pregnancy I decided everything would
be different. I enrolled in a relaxation class. I read different books on
the subject and my mind was at rest all through the pregnancy. In fact I
was on top of the world right up until I entered the hospital in labour
where I was immediately surrounded by starched frost faced sower
mouthed females who I am sure if they smiled they would crack their
faces. I was attended to by a masked cod-fish eyed female who shaved
me and gave me an enema. Whereupon she showed me into a toilet
and left the door open to add to my discomfort so she could listen to
me. By this time with enema working and my labour pains stabbing I
felt alone and wished to God I could die. After spilling half my guts into
the toilet I was then put in a bath which made me feel very hot and
giddy. Nine hours later I had my baby after a lot of screaming with the
pains I would not wish a dog to have. My baby was put into my arms
and a soppy faced bitch with a mask on and a voice of a woman who
will never give birth to anything said to me what an awful fuss you
made about nothing. They talk to you as if you are stupid and that you
are pretending to be in pain. The woman [sic] in the African jungles
have none of this to put up with. They are surrounded by their own
happy people. One good solution I think would be to have men to deliver our babies. While I attended antenatal it was men in attendance
and they were very kind and very understanding. . . . The nursing profession is very much over rated. . .I also wish that you could give birth
to a big fat nine pounder. Then I would like to read your impressions.

No Response.

CMAC:PP/GDR/D.34

Correspondence 33

May 8, 1950
Florida

Dear Sir,

This is the first opportunity I have had to write you of the birth of my seven weeks old daughter, Baby G.

The Reader's Digest's first article about your method introduced me to one of the greatest and most enjoyable episodes in my life. I wanted to write you before the baby came but could find no local doctor who followed your method. I finally found Dr. _____ who is an osteopathic doctor and let me remain at my home for the birth. I obtained your book and read it with interest three months before the baby was due. I understood everything except the relaxation but I practiced as well as I could. Baby G was two weeks overdue. March 21st, I awoke at quarter of six with contractions every seven minutes. Baby G is my second baby—I have an 18 and 1/2 month old son, Infant B, who was born in the hospital with great suffering and fear. The doctor finally put me out and applied lower forceps and episiotomy and told my husband he had saved me about four hours of pain. Infant B was several hours old before I even saw him and then the nurse just held him up about three feet from the bed and refused to let me touch him.

Anyway, we called Dr. _____ about 7:30 a.m. and he came out to check me. He said he'd leave his instruments to be boiled and be back about noon to check again, but it would probably be late afternoon or evening as I hadn't even begun to dilate yet. My husband was with me—at 10:30 the baby changed position and the first show came. We are three blocks from a phone and as the contractions came closer my husband fanned me and made me relax each time I would start to tense. I breathed deeply and then slept in between contractions. At 11:45 the head crowned. My husband asked if he should go phone since he didn't know what it was. I said 'no' because the doctor said he would be there at noon. At five minutes to twelve Baby G was born. [My husband] caught her and she cried by herself after her head and shoulders were out. The doctor came 35 minutes later and was amazed and he cut the cord, expelled the after birth and cleaned the very small amount of blood. Baby G was clean and all in all it was a very beautiful experience and one I'm sure my husband enjoyed as much as I did.

CMAC:PP/GDR/D.116

Baby G was 8 lbs. 4 oz. She is as bright and strong as a four month old baby. Everyone comments on her in comparison with other babies. I'm nursing her, of course, and having much more milk and better health than I did with Infant B.

If you write another book may I suggest a theory in which you might be interested. It is that if more mothers nursed their children they would put more time and love on them and get better results. So few mothers nurse their babies it is no wonder the children can't feel close to them—they've been pushed away from their rightful possession and can hardly expect to be as satisfied and healthy as children who are fed the way nature and God intended. Besides a normal mother enjoys the closeness with her child that nursing brings.

I want to thank you for your part in this and I assure you it was a large one. I hope your book will reach more and more potential mothers.

Sincerely,

12 June 1950

Dear Mrs.,

Your letter has arrived at long last. I was delighted to be able to add it to the many hundreds of letters that I have had from all over the world, for it is such stories of childbirth which have prompted me to continue this work for the last thirty years, in spite of the astonishingly ignorant antagonism of the medical profession. It is the women who matter, and not those who are supposed to know more about childbirth than the women themselves.

Many of my husbands are present with their wives, and knowing what they feel about it I am quite sure that your husband now will tell you that he would not have missed it for anything. It is undoubtedly true that the interference that you had with the first baby might have been avoided with a little more knowledge of the normal conduct of labor.

The fourth page of your letter is interesting for a book is just about to be published in which I lay great emphasis on the points that you raise. About a year ago a contribution of mine was published in the British Medical paper called 'The Lancet,' in which I gave the statistics of the last 500 cases that I had attended, and they showed that 98.1% of women who have natural births and are not interfered with unless it is to relieve any pain that they may have had, feed their babies from the breast. You are quite right—it is the mother-child relationship that matters in the long run—and it is on that the family unit, the home, the community, and the happiness of nations will ultimately depend.

I do not know whether you have heard of the Child-Family Digest. It is an excellent magazine, which is published monthly at a low cost, and I think you will find in it a lot of information written by some of the first experts upon this subject. . . .

My best wishes to you and your husband, and may your children prosper.

Yours sincerely,
Grantly Dick Read, M.A., M.D., Cantab.

Correspondence 34

Letter written to "Parents Magazine" and forwarded to Dr. Read.
4 May 1954
London

Dear Madam,

After reading letters in 'Parents' regarding Natural Childbirth and having heard a talk on 'Woman's Hour' by Dr. Grantly Dick Read, I feel I must write to you.

I am a disillusioned mother who has discovered through bitter experience that relaxation during labour is very difficult, and can only be achieved for a limited period of time if at all.

I feel the mother[s] who say they had an easy time through reading Dr. Grantly Dick Read would have had a comparatively easy time anyway, or have had the way paved by previous pregnancies. I have used him too!

I embarked on a first pregnancy age 20. Having read of the wonderful effects of relaxation I joined classes as soon as I gave up work. I found the classes helped me to lose most of my nervousness, and when labour started I was thankful the discomforts of waiting were over and went off confidently to hospital.

My experience, and that of the two mothers whose babies were due next, was that the breathing seemed to lessen the pain for awhile but afterwards partly due perhaps to exhaustion things got beyond us. After 20 hours I was given gas and air which, though seemingly ineffective at least gave me something to concentrate on in the nightmare that followed. An x-ray after 35 hours showed there was room in the pelvis for the child to pass but after another 5 hours it was decided to do a C-section operation to save the child, whose heart was failing. I was relieved to be told the child would be saved to know it would be born that evening, but it will always be a profound regret to me that my little daughter was not born naturally. _____ aged 25 was in labour 33 hours and had a forceps delivery, _____ aged 31 was in labour 60 hours and had a forceps delivery, the baby only just surviving.

For interest, my normal measurements are ht. 5'9", bust 37", hips 41", waist 27", weight 11 st! My baby weighed under 9 lbs.

I am sure there is some truth in Dr. Read's theories, but is it possible to wipe away the effects of generations of civilisation in a few months?

CMAC:PP/GDR/D.35

My cousin had her first baby all in the space of 2 hours, my sister in law had a baby by extended breech without needing a stitch neither knew of Dr. Read or relaxation during labour.

Another thing whilst writing is the question of breast feeding. I was absolutely confident of being able to feed my baby. Inability to do so was unheard of in the family. The second question I asked when I came to was whether you could feed your baby after a C. 'Yes dear' was the reply: but I couldn't. It just wasn't there! Everything was done to remedy the deficiency but without effect yet when I open my clinic card I see 'If you are healthy and *want* to feed your baby you *can* do so.'

What driffle, and how frustrating!

Yours faithfully,

P.S. My apologies for writing at such length!

21 June 1954

Dear Mrs.,

I am so sorry that your interesting letter of the 4th May has remained unanswered. . . .

The points in your letter that attract my attention are firstly that you were ever allowed to suffer in the manner you describe. I think that childbirth, like everything else, must be properly attended to and properly understood to get anything like a good result, and I so frequently have to sympathise with women who write to me telling me that everything went wrong and everything was dreadful and quite naturally they do not accept the fact that anyone can have a baby nicely.

If we look at the matter quite carefully and sensibly we see first of all that you have got to carry out the procedures of my teaching otherwise you can't expect to get the results. Secondly, you have got to be in a hospital where they assist you to carry it out, and thirdly but most important, you must have a doctor whose method of carrying out everything, before, during and after labour, is when I say modern according to the methods which have proved to be most successful.

And even then allowing all that, as I quote in every writing there are just three percent of women who just do not seem to be blessed by the Almighty with the ability to have their babies naturally as obviously they were intended to. When you write, 'I am sure there is some truth in Dr. Read's theories' I think you are very generous after your own experiences, but at the same time you must realise that ninety seven percent of all women who carry out these procedures correctly (and I am not talking just England but every country in the world, there are hundreds of thousands of them,) do get a result which is infinitely better than that which is obtained by those who are neither properly prepared nor looked after.

I am not criticising your doctor or yourself, I am just giving you the plain facts as I have seen them in the last fifteen or twenty years. All I can say is that I do sincerely hope that those of your family who are going to have babies in the future will make every effort to learn carefully the means by which they can get some assistance if not be completely freed of all distresses and discomforts that arise in people not quite properly made for the job.

My best wishes to you and thank you for writing a very interesting letter.

Yours sincerely,
Grantly Dick Read, M.A., M.D., Cantab.

Section 6

Feelings of Failure in Natural Childbirth

"But where did I go wrong?"

*P*erhaps the most poignant letters in the collection are those in which women express feelings of failure for not accomplishing all that Dick-Read set them up for in his writings. By writing that childbirth was a natural function, he eliminated women's choice and substituted one set of dogmatic rules (those of the scientific medical profession) for another set of dogmatic rules (those of Dr. Grantly Dick-Read). In this section the letters illustrate that one of the least attractive features of Dick-Read's writings was that it removed the uniqueness of each woman's experience in childbirth. When Dick-Read established the "norm," many women sought this avenue, and when they failed they believed that they were not normal. Correspondent 35 wrote to Dick-Read that her doctor told her that some women could achieve natural childbirth and some could not, but those that were able to would do so without Dick-Read. By this point in the volume, we should not be surprised that Dick-Read took this as an affront. When women did not achieve the natural childbirth of their expectations and wrote to him, he would respond that it was their lack of preparation or the interference of their physicians, and repeatedly urged women to have another child as soon as possible using his methods.

Correspondence 35

March 28, 1950
Massachusetts

Dear Dr. Read,

I have recently survived a natural childbirth in Boston and I would like to tell you about it in the hope that you would be willing to tell me (1) why it was such an ordeal and (2) what can be done about enlightening the obstetricians and hospitals in Boston.

I think one reason I was so eager to have a third baby was to experience a natural childbirth. My last baby was a rooming-in baby, and I felt that this would be the final step toward a fully satisfying experience for myself and the baby. I knew that my doctor 'did' natural childbirths so when I told him of my desire he said 'Fine. I think you will be a good candidate.' 'Well, Doctor, how do you feel about Dr. Read's book?' His reply was lengthy but its general substance was that Dr. Read's book was full of a lot of poppycock; and there were some women who could have a natural childbirth and some couldn't; that it was a question of psychological make up and that the ones who were naturally right for natural childbirth generally sailed through without even having heard of Dr. Read while those who were very earnest about the exercises were generally tense and nervous anyway and had a very hard time. In this whole attitude I saw an unwillingness to concede anything to you and I expect this attitude widespread.

I found your book terribly exciting and completely convincing. (The book I speak of is 'Childbirth Without Fear'.) Its great service to me was to remove all conscious fear. For nine months I looked forward eagerly to my labor. However, since I am by nature lazy, one of your negative mothers I expect, I was willing to go along with his theory that exercises were unnecessary. I also felt that since it was to be my third that my muscles ought to be sufficiently stretched to accommodate the baby. However, I became very familiar with all the stages of labor. . . .

I came to term and had strong, regular, but short lived contractions for 36 hours before I went to the hospital. Consequently, when the contractions started for the last time I was reluctant to go to the hospital until I was sure they would continue. (My doctor urged me to wait until I was sure, also.) I had a drive of half an hour to get to the hospital. The contractions during it were five minutes apart, and strong and I

CMAC:PP/GDR/D.105

found it impossible to relax then or in the hospital while I was being prepared and given an enema. The doctor had two other patients in labor and was unable to stay with me (I doubt if he would have anyway.) but came in periodically for rectal examinations and to listen to the fetal heart. An inexperienced student nurse was left with me whose chief function was to listen to the fetal heart every ten minutes and chat. You can see that relaxation under these conditions was difficult. I was offered hands to grip and the nurses were astonished to find me refusing the hands and trying to relax. After two hours of this the doctor decided to speed me along by rupturing the membranes, so I was taken to the delivery room. I was in considerable pain with every contraction all this time. I learned afterwards that the baby was in posterior position and this was the reason perhaps for all the rectal examinations. The membranes were ruptured, and a nurse was stationed on either side of me, my knees were drawn up and held by the nurses, hands given me to pull, I was told I was in the second stage and instructed to push. And I pushed! I maintain that I had no fear, but I had intense pain. I was offered anesthesia but I'm a stubborn creature and was determined to see it through. The doctor's little finger was manipulating in my rectum most of this second stage and I guess he was trying to turn the baby around. The baby finally got turned around and then I felt the head going. This *was* frightening because the doctor was washing and didn't come to do anything. Finally he came and the head was born and then the shoulders wouldn't come and then he said I must really push. He made a small incision and the shoulders came. He held the baby up and I saw him, then it looked to me as if he pulled the placenta out. I asked to see it so he held it up, remarking that it was a thing of no beauty. I felt a relief that it was over, but where was this glorious elation? Completely missing. Even when they gave me the baby to hold. Before I close this part, the baby weighed nine pounds five ounces. Could this large size have anything to do with my pain? I assure you that it was very real pain. My feelings toward you were hardly charitable at the time (most unjust of me, and I apologize) and I swore then that I would never do it again, but now I feel differently and want to learn how I can be more successful next time. Would you be willing to tell me why you think this birth was such a flop by your standards? I would also like to know if you know of any doctor in Boston who is capable of taking a patient successfully thru a natural childbirth. As far as I know, and my knowledge is very limited, there are only two doctors who are willing for their patients to try it. There was an article in Time, our leading news magazine in this country, this month quoting the head of Boston's leading obstetrical hospital, Boston Lying-In where

I was delivered, as saying that natural childbirth was a fad. In short, Boston is completely unsympathetic. I don't know what I, a layman can do to better this situation, but perhaps the best way would be to find a really sympathetic doctor, and have a successful natural birth.

This is a very long letter, and if you have read this far I appreciate your patience. I hear via my friend, Mrs. _____ _____, that you are coming to this country. I hope you will come to Boston and put some sense in their heads.

Sincerely yours,

5th April 1950

Dear,

I read your letter which arrived today with great interest and not a little resentment. For one who has the ambition to work as you worked, and the desire to perform as you desired, I consider that you had a most unhappy experience, but when I read that the doctor whom you approached to take care of you expressed the opinion of my work that you record I know from past experience that your chances of an enjoyable childbirth were minimized before your labor commenced. You did have a large baby certainly, and if it was a posterior presentation it does necessitate that discomfort by which nature warns us of abnormality. I cannot of course comment upon the labor or its conduct, for apart from being easy to be wise after the event, it must be remembered that I was not present either to observe or to correct the indications for treatment during your prolonged struggle. Perhaps I can summarize best by saying that much that you told me is certainly not in keeping with the teaching that I endeavor to communicate to students and other medical men, and perhaps it would be wisest to leave it at that.

I have heard that the Boston obstetricians are running an antagonistic publicity campaign against natural or physiological childbirth. There may be several reasons for this. Their neighbors, gained considerable acclamation, not only in America but in foreign countries, for the application of what they term 'Readism'. Secondly, it must be remembered that there is much less drama in the physiological birth for the medical man, and there is less opportunity for demonstrating his brilliance upon a conscious woman than upon one who is unconscious. Again, it may require a certain amount of patience and understanding of the phenomena of natural labor, and possibly in a case like yours more time is required to get the best results. These two reasons may be responsible for the Boston activity, but we cannot be concerned with the antagonisms of those who do not try, for the reports of those who do try are the only ones that have any value, and from all over the world, not only in America, such reports are enthusiastic, and the statistical results produced by institutions where these measures have been adopted show that they have a real advantage over the older and so-called orthodox methods. We might as well ask a vegetarian how she enjoys roast beef and Yorkshire pudding as to invite this Boston group to give their opinion upon physiological obstetrics. I know quite well that if you could have placed yourself in the hands of such men as Professor _____, Dr. _____, Dr. _____, of Yale, or many others who are a little more distant from you, the story of your labor would have been very different. If you design to have a larger family, which I sincerely hope you do, do not be impressed by the misfortune that attended your choice of obstetrician, and by the size or presentation of your baby.

I read with interest that you are a friend of Mrs. _____ _____, a lady whom I have never met personally, but whom I count amongst my friends and further one to whom I believe in due course American women will owe a very deep gratitude.

My best wishes,

Yours sincerely,
Grantly Dick Read, M.A., M.D., Cantab.

Correspondence 36

4 August 1953
London

Dear Dr. Read,

I have just found your address in the telephone book, but am not quite sure if you are the doctor who wrote 'Revelation of Childbirth,' or even if I will have the nerve to post this letter, but here goes.

I had my first baby, a boy, in 1944, when I was 18. Labor was short, only 2 1/4 hours and I had an anesthetic toward the end. It wasn't a pleasant experience, I was very ignorant and frightened and looking back, it was very painful. I came round after he was born and the nurse told me it was a boy but I wasn't very interested or pleased—didn't even like him very much!

Then in 1947 I had my little girl. I meant her to be a model baby, I read and re-read your book and tried to learn how to relax, and told my doctor that I didn't want any anesthetic. In fact I thought it would be a complete walk-over! I was very well and happy all through the pregnancy and set off for the nursing home at 2:30 am one cold November morning absolutely full of beans! But do you know, it wasn't a walkover ! I thought it would be so quick, with the first one being so quick, and I pushed away for hours. Then nurse told me to stop pushing and relax as it was only the first stage. The pains were really awful, and I was horrified and felt cheated, and had an overwhelming desire to escape. Then about 8 am I simply had to push, the doctor hadn't arrived so my daughter arrived without an anesthetic but with a great deal of noise on my part at 9:00 am. She was a darling, I held her in my arms straight after the cord was cut and felt glad I'd been conscious when she came and was very happy. But where did I go wrong?

Now I believe, after 5 1/2 years that I am pregnant again and both my husband and I are very pleased. It will be a strictly economical baby, no expensive nursing home this time, I want to stay home with a midwife or maybe my doctor to attend. But I do want to know what I can do so that I can enjoy it more. . . .I know I'm a rather nervous type of person, and I don't think I really mastered the art of relaxation, but you see I feel full of doubt, is it impossible for me to have painless labour! I definitely don't want an anesthetic, that is out, altogether, I wouldn't miss those first few glorious minutes for any amount of pain.

CMAC:PP/GDR/D.41

I know it's very bold of me to write to you like this, I'm not a patient of yours, and you must be very busy, but if you could spare a moment to write to me and reassure that it can be done then I'll do whatever you say and be very, very grateful.

Sincerely,

14 November 1953

Dear Mrs.,

Thank you very much for your letter of August 4 which has reached me where I am traveling in Central Africa at the present time.

It is quite obvious that you have completely the right idea with regard to having your baby, and the best advice I can give you is this.

Patience in the first stage of labour, relaxing with your contractions. Hard work in the second stage of labour, assisting your contractions and relaxing in between them, and self-control throughout.

If you are having your baby at home, nothing could be more ideal, for you are in familiar surroundings, you have your husband with you, and there should be no reason for you to be left alone.

I have never said that childbirth is 'painless' but there is no reason why it should not be a wonderful and satisfying experience for you. There is the possibility that there may be a tendency to backache towards the end of the first stage, but if you realize that this is only a temporary state of affairs, and will pass as the second stage of labour becomes established, you will appreciate that this is not real pain.

My best wishes to you, and I hope you will let me know how you get on.

Yours sincerely,
Grantly Dick Read, M.A., M.D., Cantab.

19 July 1955

Dear Dr. Dick Read,

You may remember me writing to you in 1953 and you very kindly replied from Africa where you were traveling at the time. I told you about my two children and you said you would like me to let you know how I went on if I had another baby.

Well, somehow I didn't manage to conceive until last October, but then I had a wonderful pregnancy, everything perfectly normal, I never looked or felt better in my life. I practised relaxation every day and felt perfectly happy and confident.

Then on July 1st, one week early, I had my baby daughter. I needn't go into details, the first stage was long, but I did just what you said and it was quite peaceful and uneventful and natural. But my baby, who was going to be so perfect was terribly deformed, and died three days ago, only 15 days old. She was born with a spinobifida, a very bad one, nearly the whole of her back was a jelly, and her legs were crooked and paralyzed and her head was soft and all bumps.

This is why I'm writing to you, to see if you could help me understand why or how. My doctor tells me to have another one, but dare I! Maybe I shall see it in a more reasonable light in time, it has been such a strain watching her die, she had such a strong heart and it went on and on even though she had no food and the last three days couldn't even swallow water or her sedative.

I should be very grateful for any advice you can give me.

Yours sincerely,

27 July 1955

Dear Mrs.,

Thank you for your letter of July 19. As I read the first page and a half I was getting so pleased with what you had written and then I came to the end of the letter. I can only offer you my sincere and deepest sympathy.

The deformity of a baby is one of the tragedies of mothers' lives. Unfortunately there is always a certain percentage and usually the cause is entirely unknown to us. In all forms of life there are accidents of development, but the reason for them is obscure.

To me both medically and philosophically, I find it a shock and a frustration which challenges both my biological and ethical beliefs. However, I can only offer you this consolation, and it is that to have this tragedy more than once is a most unusual and very rarely recorded event. I suggest strongly to you that you should put this down somehow in your mind along the lines of the ancient philosophers who upheld the view that affliction and sorrow were means by which the strength and nobility of a worthy mind were uncovered and made clear, not only to the one inflicted but to those who are around her in her normal and everyday life.

My best wishes, and I can urge you that whilst you have youth and strength to complete your family as if this had never happened, in the belief that you have not justified two such tragedies.

Yours sincerely,
Grantly Dick Read, M.A., M.D., Cantab.

Correspondence 37

August 6, 1953
California

Dear Dr. Read:
   . . . My doctor, though very sympathetic to my private attempt to follow your method, did nothing very active to help me. I had one half dose of Demerol and a rectal Nembutal and never woke up! They gave me gas, I believe at the delivery at 10:47 pm. So you see I did not do you proud and am sorry.

Sincerely yours,

2 September 1953

Dear Mrs.,
   I am glad to hear that you now have a lovely baby in spite of everything, but am very sorry you were unable to experience its birth as you had desired. However, if and when you have another child perhaps you will have better luck.

Yours sincerely,
Grantly Dick Read, M.A., M.D., Cantab.

CMAC:PP/GDR/D.103

Correspondence 38

29 May 1956
Wallasey

Dear Doctor,

Your secretary tells me that you would be pleased to hear from me, and I am so relieved, I was afraid that you might not want to be bothered with a stranger.

I very much want your advice about having a baby, but had better begin at the 'end,' and then go back to earlier years.

I am 38 years of age, and had my first baby on first of April last. It had to be removed with instruments whilst I was unconscious, and when I came round I was told the baby was dead, stillborn. This was a terrific shock and grief to me and I was very upset, 'dead, dead' kept repeating itself in my mind, and the whole world looked very black indeed.

To comfort me all the nurses, sisters, and matron kept telling me to 'have another,' that nothing would fill in the blank like this, and as I was 38 years of age to 'try right away,' as soon as possible and not let much time lapse. My elder sister who is a midwife also told me the same thing. I very much want a baby, although it is now nearly two months since the birth I am still horrible depressed and 'fed up.' Nothing seems to have any meaning any more, things seem all wrong, quite out of proportion to the fact that I have no baby when I expected one. My midwife sister tells me that this is nature urging me on, telling me to hurry to replace the missing baby, and that all my odd feelings, nervous shaking etc. will go once I am pregnant again. There is nothing I would like better but for one thing, I AM SCARED STIFF of trying again.

Now to go back to the beginning so that you may understand better. As a schoolgirl of 12 or thereabouts I was always terrified of the idea of childbirth, it assumed proportions of a nightmare to me, and having a baby always loomed up in my mind as one of the most dreadful fates which could befall me. I was so scared at the possibility of this that I made up my mind never to get married. I waited until I was 32 before getting married, and then I told my husband-to-be about my fears and he agreed to leave the choice to me, that he would never press me to have children. About this time a lot of extra work fell on me at the office, one of my sisters was seriously ill, and the combined worries gave me a batch of 'unreal feelings,' and nervous symptoms. I saw a

CMAC:PP/GDR/D.50

psychiatrist, told him of my fears of marriage and childbirth, and he told me that it was right to get married as by following nature's normal way I would come to no harm. To ignore my feelings as far as possible and follow normal instincts. Well I got married, and kept on my job for two years so we used contraceptives to avoid pregnancy.

Finally it was not necessary for me to work any more, and I had also realized how much my husband would like children, although he never tried to urge me in any way. But I felt ashamed of being such a coward, and told him he could stop using anything and 'try for a baby.' It was two years before I became pregnant.

I had read your book, 'Childbirth Without Fear,' which I read thoroughly, I attended relaxation classes at the local maternity home, and was also told to read a little booklet costing 9d., 'Relaxation and exercise for natural childbirth,' by Helen Heardman.

I did the exercises in the book which were the ones we did once a fortnight at class, and tried to relax 15 minutes every day as instructed.

When the time came for the baby to be born, it was three weeks overdue, and I had been having odd pains off and on for several weeks. I finally went into the maternity home at 11 p.m. Saturday night, I was prepared in the usual way and put to bed with two tablets, I was promptly sick and lost the tablets, but got no others. The pains in the back sickened me and although I tried to relax I found it quite impossible to do so, and gave up attempting it. Some hours later I got an injection, and later again the Gas and Air machine, but didn't seem to get a great deal of help. I was alone for most of this time. Then about 6 a.m. the following morning I went into the labour ward, and was still there about 11:30, and finally was 'put to sleep' and the baby removed with instruments. All my 'pushing and shoving' didn't appear to move it. I was in constant pain although with Gas and Air, and took the stuff to send me asleep with extreme gratitude.

PLEASE Dr. Read, what went wrong? Why was I unable to benefit from my relaxation and exercises, and why did I crack up at the first pain? Is it something wrong which I did, I thought I had practiced faithfully, but was quite unable to relax when the pains actually started.

You now see what my problem is, I want to have a baby now, not just for my husband but for myself as well. Carrying the last one roused my dormant maternal feelings, I long for a baby but am so terrified of going through 'all that again.' It is affecting my nerves, I wake up every morning with the thought 'Shall I or shan't I,' on my mind, the conflict of whether to try again or not is tearing me apart.

Common sense, doctor, and nurses, all say 'try again,' and I realize that my nervous symptoms probably come from thwarting nature, but my fear is so great. Please can you help me, can you give me some advice, details of how to relax properly or something. During my pregnancy I found great comfort in reading your book, but now that I 'failed the test' all my hope and confidence seems to be gone. Everyone says that the only way for a woman who has lost a baby to recover peace of mind is to have another, and I want another, but my fear is so great that I feel between the 'devil and the deep sea.' If I refuse to 'try again,' I will be ashamed of myself for life, and probably become 'nervy,' besides knowing I am letting myself and my husband down.

Will you please help me, and thank you very much for letting me write to you in the first place. I had just lost my baby when I read in the papers about your making a record of the birth of a baby, and envied that woman terribly.

Yours sincerely,

2 June 1956

Dear Mrs.,

I must say that I was very grieved indeed to hear of your childbirth experiences and the thoughts that had previously gone through your mind in relation to having babies.

Now that I have given up practice I like to be of what help I can to women like yourself who have suffered unnecessarily in their just efforts to become mothers. You ask me what went wrong. Well I am not in a position to tell you that except from what you write to me concerning the manner in which your labour was conducted, one might suggest that there are methods which would probably have been more helpful to you.

But it is your fear of having another baby. When you write, 'I am scared stiff of trying again,' that occupies my attention. Of course, we all know with a woman of 38 or 39, there is no reason why she should be scared stiff particularly if she has already had one baby whether it survived the birth or not, but it is poor comfort to tell a woman not to be frightened when she is frightened, and it is equally poor comfort to tell her that she can get over the cause of her fears if she embarks on them all again.

I think that is the worst possible way to go about it. What you have to do is to learn the real truth and to understand exactly why you have ever got into this state. Your body seems all right to me, but you must have your mind straightened out. It is not a very bad thought and it is one that should easily be straightened out by the right sort of doctor who understands sympathetically the complications that can arise through misunderstanding childbearing.

There is a doctor in London who sees my patients for me when they are in this condition, but there ought to be one also [where you live] . . . .I don't think you necessarily require any treatment of the mind, but just a full unraveling of your difficulty by a sympathetic man. My advice to you is try and find such a person in your area, and ask him whether he can be of help to you. The Matron of the General Hospital would probably be the best woman to see, and if not go to the Medical Officer of Health and put your case to him just as plainly as you have put it to me. If I can be of any help by giving you a letter of introduction or word of advice, I shall be pleased to do so.

My best wishes,

Yours sincerely,
Grantly Dick Read, M.A., M.D., Cantab.

Section 7

Success In Natural Childbirth

"I am delighted to be able to say that I had a natural pain-less childbirth."

Doubtless, the letters that make up this section provided Dick-Read with the greatest amount of professional pride. Looking beyond the obvious glorification of Dick-Read, these letters provide further evidence of women's childbirth experiences. Women who attempted to assert their wishes during childbirth were often ignored. For his part, Dick-Read responded to these letters in a paternalistic, congratulatory manner. He derived a sense of accomplishment and justification for the years of writing and battling the scientific medical community to make his natural childbirth procedure the established method for all women. Dick-Read developed his following by not ignoring women and, instead, validating their experiences. In his responses to the women who wrote of their success, he was a knowledgeable and sympathetic, albeit anonymous friend who was interested in every detail of their pregnancies and labours.

Correspondence 39

11 May 1946
Dorset

To: Dr. Grantly Dick Read
Dear Sir,

I am absolutely unknown to you, but feel I must tell you I have followed your teaching during my second pregnancy. My first child born 5 1/2 years ago was three weeks overdue. Brow presentation, persistent posterior, weight 8 lbs 9 1/2 oz.

After her birth I gradually put on more and more weight and had only scant periods, in March 1945 these ceased and consulted my doctor who said it was pregnancy. This I told him was very unlikely anyway he convinced me it was. In July and August I had a show my doctor giving injections against a miscarriage. In October I said to him if this is a baby it is dead. He replied if it will give you any satisfaction come in to the hospital and we will x-ray, this I did only to be told it was not a baby. Can you imagine what a shock this was. Baby was supposed to be coming in November.

I consulted Mr. _____ who told me I had gland trouble caused through my difficult confinement and also there was a baby eight weeks which made the date of it being expected sometime in May.

All through my pregnancy I have had wretched sickness.

After consulting Mr. _____ I decided to change my doctor. I came to the _____. He put me on thyroid tablets.

I had the good fortune to purchase one of your books. Practiced your exercises of relaxation and have just had the most marvelous confinement. When I arrived at this hospital with my own nurse I found the sister in charge is a very keen follower of yours, she helped me tremendously.

Tuesday morning I wakened at 3:30—pains every 25 minutes, relaxed and slept in between, at 10:20 they came every 7 minutes. I bathed, I dressed, having a light lunch at 1 o'clock my husband rang my nurse and doctor. We arrived there at 3 o'clock. Mr. _____ gave me an examination and said he would come back in the evening. Strange to relate the pains were less frequent had in fact stopped.

At 6:45 my membranes ruptured and I had a show at the same time the pains became worse I went into the labour ward I could still relax at intervals. It was not until a few seconds before baby was born that I would take a few whiffs of gas at 7:45 my own nurse delivered the baby, doctor and Sister having left the ward for a few minutes. Before the cord was cut I asked if I could see my baby. Nothing in my life has ever given me greater satisfaction. Baby G 6 lbs 8 ozs at four days old she is feeding well from the breast. My age is 36 years.

Please accept my sincere thanks.

Yours faithfully,

14 June 1946

Dear Mrs.,

Thank you very much for writing me the very interesting letter that I have just received. I do congratulate you that all your troubles should eventually have resolved in such a happy experience.

I am glad to read that the sister-in-charge follows the principles that I advise. I hear frequently from all parts of the country that the sister-in-charge of maternity hospitals or the labour wards in hospitals, approach childbirth as a physiological process so relaxation, exercises and education that I advise is being widely taught and the manner of conducting labour as I teach, both in the nursing and medical journals as well as in books, has become the routine practice after it has been once tried. I do not suppose more than one in twenty, at most, of the women who have benefited from this think of writing to me, but a day rarely passes without a letter from someone expressing gratitude that such simple measures can give such satisfactory results.

If you are at any time communicating with the sister at the _____ Hospital I should like you to tell her that I am always ready to discuss with her any points in either preparation or during labour that she finds a little difficult. I do not view this gospel that it appears to have been my responsibility to preach with any pride, but rather as a service to the women of our time and, I hope, for all time, therefore, when I can be of help I am only too pleased to offer this service.

Thank you again for your kindly letter. My best wishes to you and your small baby.

Yours sincerely,
Grantly Dick Read, M.A., M.D., Cantab.

Correspondence 40

April 25, 1947
Florida

Dear Sir:

I guess this will be one of the many letters you will receive from gratified mothers but I feel I must write you and thank you for your wonderful book.

I have a baby 3 months old, when I conceived him it was my 4th pregnancy. I had 3 miscarriages and I premature girl who only lived one and a half hours after 3 days of labor, the fact that I was to be a mother again pleased me very much. I always believed that a woman's greatest role in life is motherhood and that children are the most solid foundation to a happy congenial married life but. . . I was scared, my fears were loosing my baby, dying in child birth and having a long painful labor as I had with my other baby.

Fortunately I had a normal healthy pregnancy but in the last month my nerves got a hold of me and the nearer my time came the more frightened I got.

One Sunday afternoon my husband found in the Philadelphia paper an article about your work. He had already read it and gave it to me. I read the head lines and said root [sic]. . .childbirth is painful and nobody can tell me different but for some reason I went ahead and read it. . . about a week before my boy was born.

By the time I went to the hospital I had forgotten all about it. I was taken when my water bag broke but I had no pain of any kind for 5 hours then all of the [sic] sudden when my pains started I started remembering what I read about your article and started to think only in the pleasure I would have when they would lay my baby in my arms and wondering whether it would look like his father or I. I had taken a book with me and stard [sic] reading it when the Dr. came in to see me he immediately brought the stretcher before I knew it I was in the delivery room and had him. I kept talking to the two Drs. and nurse. I really made a nucsause [sic] of myself telling them it just had to be a boy——

All I had was 45 minutes of labor and I enjoyed that grand miracle of nature. I think the most beautiful thing I ever saw in my life was the first

CMAC:PP/GDR/D.100

time my baby smiled—no need to say he's a big, healthy contented little boy.

Thank you in the name of all the mothers who have read your book and have been influenced by it to a happier, healthier childbirth.

God bless you,

No response

Correspondence 41

11 October 1948
England

Dear Dr. Read,

Having recently joined the ranks of happy mothers who owe so much to you, I must write to thank you.

When my husband and I had been married six months we decided to have a child and were delighted when we knew there was one on the way. As you state, we couldn't believe that such a perfect sequence of events could lead to an unpleasant experience for me and as the books I had glanced at told me of so many things that could go wrong during pregnancy I asked my doctor to recommend something to me. He immediately told me to obtain 'Revelation of Childbirth,' both my husband and I read it carefully and with great interest, and I practiced relaxing although never for any length of time and had no instruction. I had placed myself in the care of Dr. _____ and visited him at the ante-natal clinic attached to the _____ Hospital . . . .Many of my friends had their babies under his care and I had the greatest confidence in him.

The nine months of my pregnancy were very happy ones. I had none of the unpleasant accompaniments that many women experience and led an active life, helping on the farm and cycling the whole time.

When I started to have a slight "leak" and regular twinges it was interesting to know that the baby's arrival was imminent. Having rung my doctor up and he had told me to come into hospital, my husband brought me in at 9:20 pm stayed with me until midnight and Infant B arrived at 2:00 am all in all seemed about half an hour to me and I couldn't believe that the baby had arrived. It was even difficult to believe it when he was given to me to hold, a few minutes old. I did not feel at all fatigued and after being brought back to my own room could not sleep because of lying awake and thinking of the wonder of it all and longing for my husband to ring at 6:00 am and learn the wonderful news— especially that it was a boy, which we both badly wanted. Dr. _____ said it was a perfect labour and that I was a model patient! Many of the sisters and nurses have come to ask me whether I'm the one who had relaxed and those who have not already read your book, tho' most of them have, want to borrow it. I myself have been reading it again and comparing my experience with some of the cases quoted in the book and am amazed at how many of the various aspects of my 'labour' cor-

CMAC:PP/GDR/D.16

respond exactly with those you describe in different chapters. When I came here my twinges stopped during the taxi journey and process of bathing so I was brought to my room, told to go to bed and ring if anything developed. Very soon contractions came every four or five minutes. However, I realized during them and they were quite bearable and I almost slept in between. Sometimes I thought of what was before me and with interest and certainty not fear which I had no trace of during the whole of my labour. At about 11:30, the contractions became rather painful and at the height of one there was a 'pop' and rush of fluid as my membranes ruptured. My husband, who had been sitting with me all the time heard the 'pop' and told the sister, who then took me to the labour ward. Before long the second stage started and this lasted 1 and 1/2 hours the doctor being with me less than an hour. As the stage developed so my consciousness became lower, at least I was gradually unaware of my surroundings except the doctor and sister by my side, and only aware of the terrific effort that was necessary with every contraction. There was no pain at all, only very hard work. It seemed only a very few contractions before I could feel the head crowning and my doctor gave me slightly different directions then. How quick and easy it was and what a wonderful experience.

Infant B is a lovely baby, and really looks several weeks old compared with many new born babies I have seen in the nursery. He was 12 days early and weighed 8 1/2 lbs and now at the end of two weeks is feeling very well. Tomorrow I take him home and look forward to caring for him myself.

As you will probably realize my husband has been a real partner in this great venture. He has shared my natural approach and that to me is most important. Most husbands knowing even less than their wives cause a deal of trouble.

I hope Dr. Read that this rambling hasn't wasted your time, but I had to write to you. You will understand more than I have written of what great joy my husband and I have.

And I now look forward to having brothers and sisters for Infant B and having a real family.

Again, many thanks to you.

Yours sincerely,

4 November 1948

Dear Mrs.,

I appreciated very much receiving your charming letter and feel again a strong sense of justification in this work that such messages bring to me. My publishers tell me that for every letter received upon a given subject they estimate that one hundred similar experiences have occurred for only one person in one hundred brings herself to write to an author. On this basis my files suggest that during the past few years over one hundred thousand women in the British Isles have experienced a relatively natural childbirth. Since it is only 25 years ago that a woman who said she had no pain at the birth of a child was considered abnormal and painless births were a form of obstetric abnormality, you will appreciate the change that has come over the attitude of women towards this natural and very beautiful event. I cannot receive too many letters like yours although scarcely a day passes without one arriving. You will be disbelieved by those who have been allowed to suffer but our experiences, unobtrusively communicated to young married women will bring far greater comfort than you yourself can be aware of.

I wish you all good fortune in your family life, for to have a husband who can become interested and take part, as it were, in the birth of his family is a tremendous asset for all time.

My best wishes to you,

Yours sincerely,
Grantly Dick Read, M.A., M.D., Cantab.

Correspondence 42

2 April 1950
Bucks

Dear Dr. Dick Read,
Perhaps your _____ copy of _____ will reach you about the same time as this letter; and I would like to explain that I am the Mrs. _____
_____ whose letter appears on pages _____. The Editor has been most kind and among his kindnesses was to send me your address as I have wanted to write to you ever since my baby's birth as described in the magazine Just two criticisms—that no mention is made of the fact that I didn't do the exercises, I did practice the relaxing daily—with great enjoyment and took raspberry leaf tea. Also, [my child] was born in 2 hrs as stated though the magazine's arithmetic makes it look like 3 1/2 hrs. . . . They are details really in a way—tho's the daily relaxing is *most* important.
Well Doctor Dick Read I vowed last July to write and thank you more than words can ever express for the great and wonderful work you are doing for women the world over. I am always telling people about your teachings because I do consider you have re-discovered an age-old truth which this world has forgotten—that children should be brought forth in joy and not sorrow. I know you have a lot of opposition in many quarters but feel sure you are consoled by the thoughts that the world in its blindness has always persecuted its greatest servants. Never mind, one day your teachings will be universally accepted. I hear and read about your methods. . .in papers and periodicals.
For myself, I can only say that the labour I have described was a great and wonderful experience and I think that the happiest day of my life. I looked forward to it *so* much and had prepared myself well and God in his goodness gave me ample reward. If I were well enough off financially I feel I should like to have another baby your way and have it filmed and televised as I believe others have done, as a permanent record of the truth of your words! Of course, this is impossible but if I ever *can* possibly help you any way I should be highly delighted. It was so very splendid to manage on my own.
Now may I suggest, humbly, the following thoughts: 1. I feel mental preparations should be stressed and in particular concentration practiced, as this was the most difficult part—to concentrate on relaxing. 2. Of course I had no enema and should hate to do so as it must be a

terrible interruption at a time when one is most busy; I think the bed should be prepared so that one can evacuate naturally and it can then be disposed of. 3. The breathing to be *very* much stressed.

You might like to know I had no after pains, and also that my bowels worked splendidly and I had complete bladder control; both those items were very bad with my first baby—afterwards I mean.

Next time you come to England I'd love to meet you. . . !

All good wishes to you in your splendid work—and many, many thanks once more for the greatest experience of my life. My husband [said] to take you along and was a great help to me.

Yours very sincerely,

P.S. The ancient Egyptians used a 'birth chair.' I wonder what it was like?

11 April 1950

Dear Mrs.,

I must reply to your letter to assure you that I appreciate you having sent it, for although I do receive many from very widely distributed parts of the world each one comes as a further justification for the principles of physiological childbirth. We have found with the years that it has a much deeper influence than merely enabling a woman to have her babies with the minimum discomfort and greatest possible pleasure, and its influence is showing itself upon society not only in the health of the mothers but in the development of the children. The mother-child relationship, I am sure you will realize, is the basis of a new philosophy, and when man holds in the palm of his hand the power to destroy all living creatures upon the earth there must ultimately come a time when one of two things will happen—either man will be destroyed or by mutual consent of those who are antagonistic in their ideologies destruction will be withheld. Then only one thing will be left— a world with an ideology based upon the philosophy of its purpose and manner of living. To that end the perfection of motherhood is obviously a factor of incalculable importance. I think, if you buy a new book of mine which will shortly be on the market called 'Introduction to Motherhood,' you will discover in it that considerable emphasis has been laid upon the points that you raise in your letter.

My best wishes to you,

Yours sincerely,
Grantly Dick Read, M.A., M.D., Cantab.

Correspondence 43

9 April 1951
Edinburgh, Scotland

Dear Dr. Read,

I thought I would like to write to you to thank you for the wonderful inspiration your book 'Revelation of Childbirth' was to me during my two pregnancies and confinements particularly my second.

I read your book for the first time, when my little girl, Baby G, was on the way, and I looked forward confidently to my confinement; it went well in the early stages, until an elderly midwife made some tactless remarks and I went to pieces. I was also left alone 'to get on with it,' and I am afraid I could never really get back to my earlier concentration.

I had a little gas and air—concentration on working the thing helped—because I found a little later it was empty anyway! They brought a refill, and it was most certainly a help. I was fully conscious when she arrived at 9:30 pm weighing 8 lbs 5 ozs—somehow, her arm was up, and it was born with her head and I was torn and had some six or seven stitches. She is now almost 21 months . . . .

When I became pregnant again, and on a second reading of your book, I knew you were right, and was determined to be successful this time.

I did your exercises. . . and felt extremely well and cheerful, had no sickness and looked forward eagerly to my confinement. My husband was most interested and encouraged me with the exercises.

My labour began about 3 pm, and the midwives arrived promptly to prepare the room, as I was being confined at home. They were very interested in what I was trying to do, and gave every cooperation.

The membranes ruptured at 6 pm, and the contractions were very strong and every 2 minutes. I was able to relax during them and felt no pain at all; not even when passing to the second stage; which I did without realising it until I suddenly found I wanted to push with the contraction.

The doctor, who I knew was not sympathetic with what I was trying to do and very sceptical, arrived about 4:30 pm, but I felt no need of him—I think he sensed this, as he left within a few minutes! I felt I didn't want any conflicting opinions around me.

CMAC:PP/GDR/D.31

The 2nd stage went well, hard work, but I was able to relax between and often dosed off, although I was very well aware of all that went on! The nurses thought I must be having pain and could hardly believe it when I assured them that there was none, and offered drugs, but I did not want them, as there was no pain.

My son, Infant B, was born at 8 pm, with no drugs being taken or administered, and it was the most wonderful feeling to hold him straight away in my arms and to know that I had achieved a really painless birth. He weighed 9 lbs 12 ozs, and I had no laceration. My husband was with me the whole time—I could never have done it without his understanding help and encouragement, as he knew what I was trying to do, and saw to it that my wishes were carried out. As for the nurses, I cannot speak too highly of their kindness and co-operation.

The placenta came away without help after 30 minutes and there was little loss of blood. Also my discharge stopped after 3 weeks; the only discomfort I had at all was from pains for about four days afterwards, particularly when feeding—I never had these with my first baby.

The baby fed well, but unfortunately he was put to the breast far too long on the first few days, and very sore nipples resulted. I had to express the milk and give it to him in a bottle for three days; my nipples healed well and I am glad to say that I was able to put him back to the breast and he is doing well—was weighing 12 lbs 2 ozs on 7 weeks.

I am so grateful to you for the inspiration your book gave me, and I am delighted to be able to say that I had a natural painless childbirth.

Yours sincerely,

As proud father I eagerly endorse everything my wife has said. I, too, have read your book carefully; I shared most enthusiastically the sense of exultation of achieving a painless childbirth. I had always wanted to be present at the birth of my children, and I was delighted to see this recommended in your book. In the event it proved to be one of the most wonderful experiences of my life.

I really felt that it was the most natural and proper thing in the world for me to be present. It left me with a profound admiration for my wife and a great sensation of closeness to my small son.

We both thank you again for the inspiration and happiness that you have given us—and wish you every success in the progress of your great work.

Yours sincerely,

17 May 1951

Dear Mr. and Mrs.,

On my return to Johannesburg two days ago I found your letter awaiting me. I am always grateful to have such records of childbirth from people I have never met. Yours was a particularly inspiring letter because it contains three factors of major importance. 1, the doctor was not sympathetic and indeed, sceptical. 2, a baby of nine pounds, two ounces born without unbearable discomfit, or physical injury to the mother, and 3, both husband and wife were present to realize what the Creator intended childbirth to be.

I congratulate you both and my only regret is that owing to the short-sightedness of many of my colleagues, who teach obstetrics, it is un-likely that I shall live to see the day which will surely come when the majority of parents will have experiences similar to yours. We shall then have commenced the breeding of a new race of men.

My best wishes to you both.

Yours sincerely,

Grantly Dick Read, M.A., M.D., Cantab.

Correspondence 44

November 10, 1952
Maryland

Dear Dr. Read,

Here are my promised remarks about my experience with Natural Childbirth. I turned to it for my third baby when I learned that my doctor and hospital here give very little pain relief. (My 3 have been born in 3 different places—signs of the times.) I had heard about it in magazine articles and knew of one person who had tried it successfully.

I worried during pregnancy, and it was not until my baby was actually born that I realized that it is possible to have a baby in a state of consciousness without horror. Now I look forward to my next baby (planned for Spring after next) with the knowledge that pregnancy can be a very happy period rather than being overshadowed by dread. My labor was so ridiculously easy that it hardly seems worth describing. A little slow in the morning, felt rather dopey all day, took it easy, had regular, long, strong contractions begin at 10 p.m., reached the hospital at 12 midnight, (couldn't believe I was actually in labor) and at 1 a.m. water broke, gave a few deep groans (although recall no actual pain) and the baby (9 1/2 lbs) born at 1:15. I accepted ether as I couldn't believe I was actually about to deliver painlessly, but never again as after this simple labor I hemorrhaged a good deal, received 2 pints of blood transfusion. I had done the same with my first baby—5 hour labor under amnesia drug, forceps delivery under ether, a lot of stitches. Then thought the bleeding due to all the surgical work, now believe it is just the ether. I know other people are not affected so much, but will request Novocain if any stitches are necessary for my next baby. This baby has been by far my easiest to care for, although he is so much like his brothers they will look like triplets when grown.

I have had a good many thoughts about childbirth during the past 5 years (my oldest is just 4) and as they all seem to relate to things you mention in passing in your book, I will send them along. Sorry this is not typewritten and on good paper—but if I wait for the typewriter to be repaired and materials to be assembled before writing, I will be a grandmother.

Your great discovery has, I feel, opened many avenues of thought, as all great discoveries do. Now that pain in childbirth is no longer neces-

CMAC:PP/GDR/D.111

sary, and can be removed from taboo topics, many of its implications can also be faced and [word missing] instead of being relegated to a conspiracy of silence. When people really accept Natural Childbirth I know tremendous advances in human happiness will come of themselves, others will be brought by interested people.

To begin at the beginning with babies themselves, I can confirm Freud on their memory of birth. My 4 year old saw some pictures of babies *in utero* in the book by Goodrich of Yale, pointed to where the cord entered the baby's stomach and kept repeating 'Drink milk in there.' When I told him about the baby inside me, he asked if it would 'come out the hole?. . . .'

I am sorry now my first two were not born ideally—although if it were not for drugs they would not have been born at all.

I am one of those women who will do everything to give a child a good life but who simply can't face the horrors of old fashioned labor. Unfortunately for the human race, it has seemed in the past that women intelligent enough to improve the race have lacked the courage to face labor, whereas less intelligent women have bred practically annually. The ones I really admire are those who were both intelligent enough and courageous enough to become pregnant while aware of what they were getting into—but they have been few and far between. I think you are absolutely right that fear of childbirth has been responsible for many women's remaining unmarried (often the best potential mothers [are] the old maid school teacher). It has also been responsible for the one-child family—and I know of women who have stopped all intercourse to avoid more children in this day and age. I also suspect that eventually fear of childbirth will be found to be the cause of otherwise unexplained sterility, particularly among women of high intelligence. (I am thinking now of your Royal Commission on Population Report.) A Chicago obstetrician seems to be getting warm in his thinking (Time Magazine article of last summer). He believes some sterility is due to neurosis or something—he seems to be a bit of a misanthrope. He doesn't get to what I think is the point—their troubles all stem from fear originally.

Another great improvement in the human lot will be relations between husbands and wives. I get mad at husbands—they can do no right it seems, either by worrying about their wives or by just waiting until the whole thing blows over—but they really have been in a bit of a quandary for these many hundreds of years. The Yale Clinic for Natural Childbirth has taken a wonderful step here, which you undoubtedly know about, in letting husbands stay with their wives through labor. This I think should be marvelously satisfactory all around, even including the overworked doctor.

As to the relation of mother to child, I tend to think how I would have felt about my baby if he had been born in the usual circumstances. As it is, I just simply love him—not so desperately as I love the others, but naturally and better for him and myself I feel. I think that having a child naturally uses up enough mother instinct or whatever it is so that one does not dote upon the baby or be too possessive.

Next to my own satisfaction comes my pleasure in the fact that a good friend of college years had her third baby naturally, an experience she badly needed as her second had caused her terrible suffering which she is no better equipped to bear than I am—and she has never been able to give that child the love she needs.

Among improvements that interested people will bring about, I number everything [having] to do with children. Enclosed is an article from Today's Woman for November 1952. I am firing off a letter to the Editor today, pointing out that now that women can produce their children painlessly on their own, they are in a position to demand pleasant conditions under which to do it. You have really placed a great power for good in the hands of women, and it could lead to goodness only knows what results. As to pleasant maternity hospitals, my pleasantest was in Auckland, New Zealand, where my second baby was born, at _____ Hospital. If you tour the Commonwealth and visit Auckland I hope you will give my best wishes to Dr. _____ there and the matrons and sisters at _____.

Sincerely yours,

P.S. Another angle of Natural Childbirth is the bad effect old methods have on medical people. I know my doctor dreads the labors of his patients as much as they do. (He is very nice, and comes to the hospital to give at least moral support—he still can't get it out of his head that childbirth has to be terrible even though he saw me produce a baby with no trouble.) I am sure the wear and tear on nerves of doctors and nurses sends them to an early grave. Now that I am all set, I would like to do something for them! When I told my doctor I wanted more children, he looked surprised and said he had only heard one woman say that before.

P.P.S. My comment about learning the necessary technique for having a baby comfortably is that it is easier than one would believe. In other books than yours, articles, etc., the authors stress an early start and lots of practice. Actually, I found that about 25 sessions of relaxing (using suggestions in Goodrich of Yale's book) got me to a point where I could relax quite well enough at will. Then, being pregnant and lazy, I just rested a lot, relaxed at times, resumed relaxing about a month before [the] baby [was] due. He was 6 weeks later than predicted, and several nights around his supposed due date I was awakened by pains more severe than any in my actual labor!

Undated [most likely written in December 1952]

Dear Mrs.,

I enjoyed reading your letter very much and feel that you have a great deal in common with many lines of thought that have emerged from my experiences.

I will certainly remember to give your best wishes to Dr. _____, either when I visit New Zealand or when I write to him as I may well do in the near future.

You would not wish me to take your letter point by point, I am sure, but I would like you to watch for the new edition of Childbirth Without Fear which I hope will be published early next year, and you will read in that many of the statements and suggestions that you have made.

You will realize, I am certain, the extent to which I am guided by the comments, criticisms and experiences of vast numbers of women whom I have not had the pleasure of knowing personally, but who write to me. Your letter, from that point of view, is of great value and I would like you to know once more how very much I appreciate the trouble you have taken in sending me your thoughts and observations.

My best wishes for a very Happy Christmas and New Year.

Yours sincerely,
Grantly Dick Read, M.A., M.D., Cantab.

Correspondence 45

February 13, 1953
Texas

Dear Dr. Read:

I hope that this letter reaches you someday. When I saw your letter in TIME in response to their article, 'Natural or Unnatural,' I knew that the time had come to write you. This letter is only four years late.

This is really just a personal testimonial; I don't know what is going on in the medical profession in this part of the country. But I do know for certain that I owe you a tremendous personal debt of gratitude, and I want to thank you on behalf of myself, my husband, and my children.

Four years ago there was no word in south Texas about natural childbirth. I heard of your book, 'Childbirth Without Fear' from my sister who lived with a nurse. This nurse was your first advocate that I heard about, and while she wasn't free to put your whole 'system' in practice, she found that even a touch of it with her O.B. cases was of amazing help.

That was really five years ago when I first got pregnant, and my husband and I devoured your book. Then we had to fight it out with our doctor, who at first refused to take me. He gave in when convinced that 'after all, it can't do any harm,' and he left standing orders for drugs for me at the hospital when I called for them, which he was sure I would do.

My husband was the assistant that you say each mother must have, and our experience together in labor was the final cement to an already close relationship. The hospital and the nurses did everything to frighten me, but since there were other women wailing and causing trouble in labor, and only one R.N., we were finally left alone and were able to proceed with natural childbirth. We had your book with us in the room, and my husband paged through it madly, looking up relevant passages during my labor. As you might guess, the baby was almost born in the room. I waited twenty-five minutes on the delivery table for the doctor, strapped down, under the lights, with rude nurses around me, but my husband just on the other side of the door!

Needless to say, it was a tremendous experience, but you know that part of it. I do think, though, that I made quite an impression on the doctor and the hospital. A huge fuss was made over me the next day, and I learned later (after moving away) that the doctor who had at first

CMAC:PP/GDR/D.109

refused to take me as a patient had started natural childbirth classes for his O.B. patients, with his own special nurse to go along with them in labor! And that before I saw a single article anywhere about the system.

When my second baby was expected. . .I found a doctor in sympathy with your system, though he had never seen it in practice. Thank goodness, as I had several girlfriends who had wanted to have their babies my way and whose doctors had agreed, only to 'double-cross' them at the hospital and knock them out as soon as they go there (when they were in no position to argue).

Of course, I still had to do all the studying and exercises on my own. And we had a difficult time finding a hospital where my husband would be allowed with me in labor! Then we were treated as usual when we got to the hospital! In the middle of my concentration the nurse even came in and bawled us out for moving a wastebasket in the room!! Again the baby sneaked up on us and I had to wait on the delivery table half an hour among nurses who wouldn't even talk to me. But my doctor had several doctor friends in the delivery room, doctors who had been interested in your system but who hadn't quite believed it, I guess. . . .Neither of my doctors had believed I would go through with it, and were quite astounded, as well as the nurses in the delivery room who were fascinated by the fact that I was so thrilled as the baby emerged (and with no pain), yet cried out at the stitches done under Novocain! (Proving that I was not a mere stoic.)

And what a fuss the next day! Every other nurse in the hospital must have been in to see me, asking sweet questions, many of them saying that they had been afraid to have babies, that mine was the only way, etc.

This is just a silly personal story, but I wanted to prove to you that even without clinics or medical help, natural childbirth makes a terrific impact on the individual woman, and all we need is a chance and more of us would want it. I've had a few personal converts who were successful and who have written me touching letters of thanks. I've seen both of my babies gain back their birth weight in two days! I've heard both of them cry (and doctors have commented on it) before the doctor could even tell their sex, as they weren't fully born yet! I['ve] seen them thrive after I brought them home, as fat and healthy as could be, which may be only a coincidence, but I'm the only girl I know whose babies haven't had a touch of colic!! And such happy babies! I never had a minute's trouble with either of them, though both were bottle babies.

There's not much more I can say, except a million, million thanks to you. I'm only sorry I didn't sit right down and write and thank you four years ago as I intended to do. You are doing a wonderful thing for the women of the world. Anyone who has lain [sic] in a maternity ward and heard the other women screaming and begging for a shot (that can't be given anymore or it will stop labor) understands what your system means. It's only because it's more trouble for the doctors that it hasn't become more widespread. But someday they'll discover its value. Keep on with the good work and know that you are blessed in many homes.

Sincerely,

25th February, 1953

Dear Mrs.,

I appreciate very much the letter that I have received from you.

You represent a very large group of women in the United States who are opposed by this astonishing antagonism of the medical profession to the use of common sense in obstetrics. All over the world, I have met with agreement from women, but relatively rarely have medical men had the desire to study the wishes, comforts, health or the happiness of their patients before their own convenience.

This can only be altered by the implementation of a loud, mass demand by women that this nonsense into which science has led them should be clarified. I am grateful indeed, that there are women of your caliber and understanding who have the urge to assist in presenting this cause in such a manner that in a few years it will be established as the principle of childbirth throughout the United States.

My best wishes to you, and your husband whose tenacity against odds I admire immensely.

Sincerely yours,
Grantly Dick Read, M.A., M.D., Cantab.

Correspondence 46

October 20, 1953
Alaska

Dr. G. Dick Read,
Infant B is five months old now and I do wish I could have written you sooner.

I am very happy with the way my delivery went. I had no anesthesia whatever except as the head crowned and I wish I hadn't had any then. I was doing well when the Dr. said he could see the head or some such statement and it frightened me and I asked for the mask. Before this the nurse kept trying to put the mask on my face and the Dr. told her to leave me alone until I asked for it. He is sympathetic with your system but lets each woman work it out for herself.

It is quite difficult for a person like myself to follow directions and carry them out faithfully. Therefore I was a little lax in practicing my breath [sic] control and relaxation. Believe me next time I will be more efficient.

I relaxed as best I could through the first stage and all went well. I was amazed when the second stage started, I hadn't suffered at all through the first stage and kept expecting things to get out of hand. The Dr. was in the operating room with a baby of a friend of mine and the friend was with me and we were all wondering what was taking him so long and if he would get done in time to deliver my baby. All this added to the tension and yet I think it took my mind off myself and made things easier. Like you said the transition from one stage to the other is the most nerve racking. I felt I had to move my bowels and got out of bed and started down the hall to the bathroom. They shooed [sic] me back to bed. Then the second stage started.

I called the nurse and told her and she kept telling me to relax. I couldn't understand why she should tell me this and I tried to explain that the second stage had started and I couldn't help myself, I had to push and strain. The contractions came closer and closer and finally I could feel the baby coming. The doctor was still in surgery and the nurse was still telling me to relax. I had no pain whatever only great straining. In between contractions I was dopey and couldn't focus my eyes on the light in the room. My husband was there timing my contractions and he could hardly tell when one ended and the next one began but to me it seemed 5 or 10 minutes between. The doctor finally came to see me and examined me and immediately took me to the delivery room. It was all done in about 10 minutes. The doctor announced 'It's a boy' and I heard him cry and he put him on my stomach to see. I couldn't touch him because they feared I might infect him some way. I was so happy that I began to cry and laugh at the same time. I was afraid I would become hysterical.

The whole experience was very satisfying and enthralling. Now I am one of your apostles with experience behind me. I plan on having another child in the near future and am looking forward to the experience.

A few days after the baby came my doctor and I had a long talk about the delivery and what I could do to improve. He said he was surprised when I asked for the mask. He said I did very well and was quite proud of me.

I nursed Infant B until just the other day. I could continue but I have developed a lump in my breast and the doctor thought it might have been from lactation but I have stopped and the lump is still there so I will have it looked into to be sure it isn't cancer.

Thank you for being you and giving womankind your great gift. I am so thankful for my glorious delivery instead of a terrifying experience.

Do you know some women think I am crazy when I talk about enjoying the delivery. I honestly believe they think it's not quite decent not to suffer the tortures of the damned when a child is born. Civilization is a curse.

I must close. I will write in a few years after our next child comes.

God bless you,

Undated reply

Dear Mrs.,

Thank you so much for your very charming letter of the 20th October, which has reached me in Nairobi where I am nearing the end of a survey of normal labor amongst the most primitive tribes of the continent of Africa.

I am so glad that you were able to experience a really happy birth and I do most sincerely congratulate you on your perseverance and control in face of a certain amount of skepticism. I was, however, very sorry to read that you were not allowed to take your small son in your arms the moment he was born for fear of infection. If some of these people could see what I have seen on my tour it would help so many mothers in the world today.

I was pleased to read that your Doctor had sufficient sympathy with my methods to allow you to carry them out without interference, and I shall certainly make a note of his name for other mothers-to-be who write to me from the area.

My best wishes to you, your husband and Infant B, and may you have many, many years of happy family life.

Yours sincerely,
Grantly Dick Read, M.A., M.D., Cantab.

Correspondence 47

November 1954
Surrey

Dear Sir,
    I've been listening to the Woman's Hour Program. My daughter had a baby two years ago. I wasn't there and only received her account by letter. She read your book. I wonder if you would care to read her letter. . . .
    Forgive me if its just a crashing bore but to me its a joy. I had an easy birth not so easy as this one.
    Thanks to you and its time I said thank you.

Yours sincerely,

23 October 1953
Dublin, Ireland

Dear Mummy,
    Thank you very much for the telegram, flowers and letter. Everything has been so easy, and comfortable that I don't really believe it all. I had the idea, in spite of Grantly Dick Read, that having a baby was awful agony, but that when it was over it was so nice that you felt it was worth it, or even tended to forget how bad it was. The result is that I feel it can't really have happened yet even though there is a most healthy little being in the cot. . . .
    For two or three nights I had been feeling a bit of guts-ache in the evenings, but I don't know if that is relevant, or if it was just constipation. On Tuesday night it was a bit worse than usual, but by no means anything special. _____, _____, and _____ [family friends] were in, and we had a pleasant evenings' chat. When they left, at about 11:00 I told _____[husband] I felt tired, and had a bit of a pain and I got cocoa, and a hot water bottle, and we went to bed. I told _____[husband] that perhaps I might be starting because when a pain came my tummy felt hard when I pressed it, (or at least I thought it did some times, all these nice simple medical directions are a bit too simple, after all what is 'hard'?) We decided to try and sleep and leave it over till morning. However, I only slept lightly, and at about 3 a.m. I got a rather sharp

CMAC:PP/GDR/D.38

pain, and felt sick so I lept up for the bathroom and vomited a tiny bit, and had a drink of water. I was just going back to bed when I suddenly felt wet with about a cup full of water so I presumed this was 'the water breaking' and woke _____[husband]. _____[doctor] said I was to go to the home if I got pains every 15 minutes or if the waters broke and I wet my pants. I got back into bed and poor old _____[husband] stumbled out of bed, and drove down to the telephone. He returned soon to say that the [Home] was full, but that they were finding me a place somewhere else, and [he] was to ring back in 1/2 hour. He went out again then, and they said we were to go to the _____.

We got here, and the night nurse received us. We told her the case history, and she said would I like to go to bed, or stay up, so I said being such an unearthly hour I'd go to bed. Which I did. She explained that the house staff was scanty, in fact she was the only one on duty, and that people usually had their own nurse full time, could she get one for us? So we said ok. For the rest of the night she let _____[husband] stay with me, and she put her head round the door occasionally, and we could of course ring if we had wanted her.

For the rest of the night I was almost asleep between the pains, and lay on my back and relaxed when they came. I found that if I relaxed from my toes upwards it was the final relaxing of my cheeks that really did the trick, and reduced the pain. _____[husband] time-checked, and I was shatteringly regular at 10 minutes.

When morning came 'my' nurse turned up, and she soon sent _____[husband] off. Poor boy he was in a worse state than me having been awake and up all night. I at least had been half asleep most of the time.

A digression now on Nurse. She is another _____[family friend]. She is as sensible and canny as _____[family friend], but being a trained nurse not so full of old wives tales. She is marvelously efficient, but though everything is perfectly organized, you hardly notice the organization, and there is none of this awful medical regimentation, and bussle, and starchiness. She is a kind and motherly sort, but thank heavens not soppy, and sentimental and clearly of the opinion that though babies are the most wonderful thing in the world, they should be fed, washed, and *ignored*.

To return now. I went on lying on my side half asleep, or rolling onto my back to relax when a pain came, until lunch time. Various nurses flitted in, and out, and _____[doctor] looked at me. They prodded me occasionally, and talked to me a bit, but generally they left me to myself though nurse stayed in the room all the time. The time passed quite quickly in my half awake state. Nurse said that when the pains got too bad I was to tell her, and she would give me an injection. She offered it to me several times, but I said I was ok. The pains did get bad, but far from being unbearable. I'd far rather have a baby than food poisoning, or even a bad patch of indigestion. _____[doctor] came in just before 1 pm, and asked if the pains made me bite my lip. I politely told him that I was trying to relax, and so lip-biting didn't really come into it. He looked a little taken aback. He went off then to give a lecture. Almost as soon as he had gone the pains got much less, and then I suddenly wanted to push, like spending a penny. I asked nurse if I should push, or not, and she told me to push away. At the second push suddenly woosh, the waters really broke like a Niagara. Apparently what had come before were only the 'forewaters.' All sorts of nurses were in, and out, and around, clearing the decks for action, putting a couple of boards under the mattress, and getting water, and instruments but according to instructions I tried to sleep between contractions, and push when they came. I specially call them contractions because the pain was only just enough to tell me when I ought to push, and when I pushed there was no pain at all, and between the contractions there was not pain at all. I did actually nod off for a moment and in so doing twitched, so nurse asked me if I was in pain and so woke me up.

At 2 pm they started trying to get hold of _____[doctor], but I gathered from the whispered conversations that there was someone gossiping on the telephone, and the operator would not break in.

Apparently _____[husband] rang up at 2 and was told there was 'no change' and he could come and see me. He turned up here, presumably at about 2:20 or so, and tapped at the door. He was shattered to be confronted by a rubber-gloved, masked nurse who told him it was a girl!

Meanwhile _____[doctor] had turned up in a mad rush, and just had enough time to wash his hands and get ready in time to deliver her. As soon as he took over, he told me to take chloroform, and as he was in charge, and very distracted I couldn't very well argue, so I took it. By the feel of things the head was born by the time I took the chloroform so I suppose the chloroform was to make sure I wouldn't wriggle at the wrong moment. I was only under for a couple of minutes. It was horrible coming round, but when I did I could hear Baby G bawling and they told me it was a girl and that _____[husband] was outside.

_____[doctor] poked my tummy, and the after birth came away. Then everyone cleaned up, and they let _____[husband] in at once. I felt perfectly all right except a bit empty and weak, and I greeted _____[husband] by vomiting into the bowl he grabbed—that horrid chloroform. He stayed for a bit, and then went off to send off letters and telegrams, etc.

Nurse asked if we wanted her to stay on, we had originally only asked for her for the labor. We thought we might as well do the job properly so she is still in charge, and sleeps in here, and I'm very glad she's here, because I can ignore all the yells and gurgles, and I've got nothing to worry about (Baby G stays in here all the time.)

I am the pride of the Home for having the child so quickly, and easily, and all the nurses were full of admiration for my demonstration of relaxation, and were gushing about it to each other, and to the Quack. Since she did come so quickly, and easily, she really looked like a baby right from the start. _____[husband] and I were both expecting an obscene wrinkled red sausage of a thing, after all, new born kittens and puppies aren't so good! But to our amazement she looked just like any small baby you'd see in a pram, right from the beginning. Her hair is dark, and her eyes (of course) are dark blue. I didn't think she looked like either of us, but Nurse said she looked like _____[husband], and much to my amazement I see now that he does look like her. Isn't it silly how you have no idea of what people you live with look like?

I'm afraid my maternal instinct didn't bust forth the moment I heard her cry, but now that I have felt her, and had a good look at her, and got used to her, I am beginning to get quite soppy.

I haven't got enough milk for her yet, but nurse seems to take that for granted, which is cheering. Both you and Mrs. _____ seem to have suffered from nurses who led you to believe that such things were unheard of.

Nurse promises to get Baby G so well trained before she leaves here that I'll hardly know I have her when I get home. I doubt that, but I don't think she'll be too bad.

_____[husband] had been an absolute darling all along. What with looking after me, and getting odd things, and sending messages, and looking after the house, and feeding himself, the poor boy is destroyed. And on Monday he'll have to start lectures. . . .

                                                              Lots of love,

Dr. Read writes back to the mother:
29 November 1954

Dear Mrs.,

It was very charming of you to write to me and to send me the delightful letter from your daughter. It is, as you may imagine, most gratifying to me to get such records of which, by the way, I have got some thousands from all over the world.

It is an extraordinary thing, isn't it that such a straightforward simple, common-sense affair has escaped the notice of our profession for so many years. Happily it is spreading now and women have got the good sense to demand their rights in being an opportunity of having more or less carefree and relatively comfortable labor instead of so much of this deep anaesthesia and interference.

I wish, of course, that one expert in this approach to childbirth had been looking after your daughter because she wouldn't have been given, as she rightly terms it, that horrid chloroform which made her sick, and probably actually spoilt one of the greatest joys of all, and that is the fully conscious reception of her baby in her arms directly it is born. But still, we are ploughing along and we are getting somewhere.

It is so nice to have letters from ladies like yourself who obviously appreciate the efforts that are being made on behalf of the women of our time.

When you write your daughter, give her my best wishes,

Yours sincerely,

Grantly Dick Read, M.A., M.D., Cantab.

Correspondence 48

17 January 1956
Birmingham

Dear Sir,
    Carry on with the good work.
    It is just *plain common sense*, what you are trying to teach to the people, but how many have got common sense today. The sooner we all get down to understand the ways of nature the better.
    I am a woman of 50. How I wish I could have my babies all over again with your natural methods. Fear is the root of all our pains.
    If we loved more, or would only try to understand the word Love the world would be a better place to live in.
    I cannot write any now as I have to go in the hospital for a while.
    I am only a working class woman and I could talk better to you, than write, as you can see. But I am very sincere about your work. I only had to look at your picture in the 'Graphic' to know what a nice good kind man you are. I wish I could meet you someday.
                                                            Yours sincerely,

15 February 1956

Dear Mrs.,
    Thank you very much for your letter of January 17. . . .
    I feel quite sure that with your sensible approach to the subject you are helping a great many ladies to believe as you do yourself.
    I am so sorry to hear that you had to go into the hospital, but I hope it was nothing serious and that you are now quite well again.
                                                            Yours sincerely,
                                    Grantly Dick Read, M.A., M.D., Cantab.

CMAC:PP/GDR/D.48

Correspondence 49

21 January 1956
Cheshire

Dear Dr. Dick Read,

This letter should have been written six years ago, and again three years ago, but only now to coincide with the birth of my third child, do I hear that you are possibly in this country. We have heard of you in Canada, in the United States, in South Africa, but never in the familiar places in the British Isles where we could hope to hear you lecture, or more delightful still have the chance of thanking you personally for all that your teaching has done for us.

When my first son aged 6 1/2, was in the making, my husband early bought 'Revelation of Childbirth,' on which he had his eye for some years. I can only say that we *lived it*. Altho' 28 years old I was [uninformed about] childbirth, and pregnancy, [and was, therefore] completely uncorrupted, and at the same time completely ignorant. There had been no babies in my family since my appearance, and no friends with babies and they held no interest for me whatsoever. The result was that innumerable ludicrous and horrific tales were not in my experience, but neither was any knowledge of a more suitable kind.

Thanks to our being attached to _____ University Professor _____ undertook to look after me and in response to my lengthy typed list of questions, gently suggested that I buy his 'The Childbearing Years.' With these two invaluable publications in hand we sailed through the most marvelous pregnancy. Being very tall, I was not too overburdened and continued our strenuous country life until a few hours before delivery. In fact I was transplanting a tiny rosebush, a wild one, when Infant B decided to start his journey into the world.

This delivery, identical with the second in every respect, namely 8 hours duration, baby born within minutes of membranes breaking, result 7 1/2 lb boy, alas due to slight over enthusiasm, a slight tear, was otherwise perfect. An interesting fact in both cases was, that at _____ Hospital, Manchester, where both took place, the nursing staff, Sisters, Assistant Matron and pupil midwifes, while being slightly staggered by these 'controlled labours' were absolutely thrilled and in complete sympathy, whereas the doctors apart from the 'real' men like Professor _____ and _____ _____ (I speak in confidence!) evinced only a wall-like stupidity or incapacity to assimilate.

CMAC:PP/GDR/D.51

How many times have I read in the notes submitted to you by mothers and published at the back of your book 'it was a marvelous experience' and that is the whole of it—no words can really say more.

Now I have my daughter one week old by my side and it is the same again. This time she appeared at home with the superb cooperation of the County Midwife, who was delighted with the chance of witnessing and superintending my delivery 'a la Dick Read!' This time a big girl 8 lbs 4 ozs has joined the lively family, and no tears, not even the scars touched. Friends have always commented on the fact that our children have properly defined and rather handsome features very early and we often wonder if that is a characteristic of 'your babies?'

It has interested me to find that in four out of five cases when I have made a new acquaintance up here, and decided or discovered that we speak the same language, I have also discovered that they also have followed your teaching. A small number of us here, have certainly found it impossible not to spread your gospel wherever possible, until I think, we were likely to become bores.

Here also I must apologize for my verbosity, but perhaps it may be excused on the grounds of being six years worth!

There is however one aspect of childbirth, on which I wonder, if you have also developed control theories. Namely, the emotional reaction following delivery. The first superb exhilaration, when I am quite sure one *could* get up if one tried; then the trembling and tiredness, the longing of sleep that will not come due to an excitement, reliving every phase of the delivery with pleasure, but without the capacity for relaxation. . . .

I venture to ask if you consider that there is (in addition to the physical exercises) any mental training or say emotional, for the puerperium which would benefit the trained mother?

With apologies for taking up so much of your valuable time, and the hope that one day we may have the privilege of thanking you personally.

May I add tentatively, that I think that only during confinement do I allow myself the doubtful leisure of turning introvert!

Yours sincerely,

7 February 1956

Dear Mrs.,

I am sorry you have had to wait so long for a reply to your delightful letter which I may say I appreciate your having written to me very much indeed.

Quite apart from the pleasure it gives me to hear your experiences, your views and your feelings about childbirth, you make some extremely shrewd observations. What a muddle obstetrics is in this country. Nobody is teaching it properly, nobody knows what to teach and those who believe in the natural method daren't teach it because there seems to be some taboo on it from the Royal College of Obstetricians and Gynecologists. There are those who teach it and get the most marvelous results and therefore run into that ridiculous jealousy from their colleagues which makes life almost unbearable.

I frequently think that one of the happiest decisions that I was guided to make very many years ago was that I would never become a member or fellow of any college which could alter my views or activities upon childbirth. Consequently, I decided from the beginnings to go on in my beliefs alone. This was forty years ago, and if they proved to be right, all right they would live and if they were wrong, they would die and who could grumble, and so I think there is no question that we were perfectly right in 'assuming,' now that this approach to childbirth has justified itself all over the world, even from the mouth of the Pope concerning a good Norfolk Nonconformist, which is little short of a miracle in some ways!

I think there is something in what you say about [how] these children mature, satisfied and well adjusted at an early age. An American woman wrote a long article on a series of cases and there is not doubt that the naturally born baby has both certain assets not only in the immediate present, but in the development of the future which the baby who has had interference at birth cannot be sure of obtaining.

I was very pleased to hear of Professors _____ and _____ _____. I believe they are _____ and _____ respectively. I think I have met Professor _____ _____ at Oxford some years ago, but I don't remember whether I have met Professor _____ or not.

I shall certainly look forward to an opportunity of meeting you personally should the occasion arise, but since I have been back in England I have not had Manchester on my lecture program, although I was up there before I went away, but it may be that in due course they will want to see my face again, grey and haggard though time has made it!

My best wishes to you and your husband.

Yours very sincerely,
Grantly Dick Read, M.A., M.D., Cantab.

Section 8

Writing to Dr. Grantly Dick-Read:
Special Themes

*D*ick-Read took his role as advisor beyond childbirth and corresponded on issues as diverse as marital affairs, husbands' role in childbirth, and age as a factor in successfully accomplishing the favorable results of natural childbirth. His responses were consistently a guide to motherhood. There was no exception to what he believed to be a woman's appropriate role and the normal method for accomplishing her most important mission. In the end, Dick-Read, whether giving advice on childbirth, other medical issues, or private family matters, participated in many people's personal lives. By corresponding with the people who sought him out, he adopted the role of counselor and advisor to all those who, having formed a personal relationship with him by reading his books, took the time to ask his opinions.

AGE AND NATURAL CHILDBIRTH

Correspondence 50

21 July 1949
London

Dear Dr. Dick Read,

I felt I would like to tell you how helpful and reassuring I find your book—Revelation of Childbirth. Having heard so much about it, both first and second hand, as soon as I certified pregnant, I got a copy and studied it carefully.

I am due to produce my first baby (a bit late owing to a miscarriage 2 years ago) in September at the advanced age of a month over 39, at the _____ Hospital. Even though I have always considered childbirth a normal affair and planned a family of 6 or 7 (unfortunately I haven't married soon enough to do this) your book has completely re-assured me and I am now looking forward with patience and pleasure to the birth of my already very active child.

It is a great thing that the _____ Hospital is so insistent on prospective mothers attending their relaxation and exercise classes. I think it must be difficult to do these alone especially if the people who will help one produce one's baby are not in sympathy with these aids to birth.

I only hope that at the time one is not left alone too much or too long. Especially when first experiencing such a wonderful but slightly mystifying event, one must need an encouraging hand to hold and face to see.

One thing I did not gather from your book—have you ever had a mother, for example, for her first three babies in every case found she has had a normal, quick and easy childbirth? Also have you found that mothers whose first babies come without your teaching, have come with difficulty and pain, when they subsequently have the benefit of your teaching, have all successive births with ease and comfort? I'd be rather interested for clarification on this point—

Another question—You mention the perfect brassiere you wear at the time and that a West End Store now sells it—Can you please tell me the name of the store and the name under which it is sold? I've never really found a comfortable brassiere (except one I got for 1/6 in

---

CMAC:PP/GDR/D.48

Belfast years ago and threw out when worn out—never thinking then of having it copied) and would like to have a chance of buying one that may solve my problems—and expensive experiments.

Fortunately I've been able to lead a normal life up to date in my pregnancy, had no sickness but, spasmodically, slight indigestion and heartburn. Three weeks holiday in a very [quiet] corner of Cornwall has now set me on my feet for September when one day I remarked to my husband I wished a passing car would take pity on my condition and offer me a lift up a particularly steep hill—we walked about 5 miles daily—he remarked I shouldn't look so disgustingly healthy because no one would stop for me looking as swell as I did! He's wonderful at not letting me get lazy or taking advantage of my condition.

Again thank you so much for writing your book and so letting people who aren't your personal patients share in your teaching.

By the way are you Norfolk by birth or adoption? I can claim it by birth.

Yours sincerely,

16 August 1949

Dear Mrs.,

Thank you for your charming letter. I must write and send you my best wishes and even though at so great a distance, urge you to remember the three great virtues that I attribute to the best type of mother. They are as applicable during labour as during the whole of the life of an individual and they are patience, self-control and hard work. If you remember patience during the first stage of labour and exert an understanding self-control to accept with confidence the varying sensations and emotional changes during labour of which you will become aware and finally, if during the second stage you are willing to persist in hard muscular effort to help your baby into the world, there is no reason whatever why you should not be successful in having your child according to the laws of nature, without interference with the function by either anesthesia or manipulation.

I especially hope that you will have someone with an understanding mind to guide you through the various phases. It is the greatest examination for which a woman has to sit. Not only does she succeed because of the manner of her preparation but she is enabled to succeed by the assistance given during the process. I do not know whether these procedures are practiced by everyone at the _____ Hospital. I can only hope and in due course shall look forward to hearing from you that you have been able to recognize that childbirth, although hard work which demands the concentrated best in a woman, can be the most exhilarating achievement that she can perform.

You ask me two simple questions. I have had many women who have had families of five and six children all of them completely naturally and all of them prompting the mothers to have more children because of the happiness that the birth of a child has brought to them. The second question—many of my patients are sent to me who have had very difficult first labours and have been frightened to have a second child. They are perhaps those who give me the sense of greatest responsibility for there is a background to overcome, but the large majority of them are so astonished at the difference of their second labour from the first that they have no hesitation in increasing their families.

You ask me about brassieres. There is a company in London called Decreed Products Limited, 31 Palace Street, S.W. 1, and if you write to them pointing out that you wish to obtain such brassieres as I have described they will give you any information that they have upon the matter and the retail shops from which the article may be obtained.

Yours sincerely,
Grantly Dick Read, M.A., M.D., Cantab.

23 September 1949

Dear Dr. Dick Read—

I was so glad to have your letter dated 16 August and it was more than kind of you to answer from such a distance when you must be up to your eyes in work. When I wrote first to you I'd not known that you were not in England. Your attorney however acknowledged my letter—said he had sent it on and gave me [the] address of the brassiere makers. I have one but haven't started wearing it yet. In the hospital I was in a nursing one.

I am now the proud relation surprised possessor of a son, born 7 September—7 lbs 15 oz—I thou't I'd have a daughter somehow. My husband's terribly proud of him—thinks he's a fine child. Luckily the child returns the compliment and finds being held and talked to by father most reassuring and comforting.

In the end, rather unexpectedly, I had a Cesarean Section. I went to the _____ Hospital on Tuesday, 6 September, with regular first stage pains about 8:30 pm and they expected the baby by breakfast next day. However, I made little progress in the night or during the day till tea time when I did put on a bit more speed and the pains gradually changed more to second stage. I really suffered little discomfort and was quite happy. However at 7:30 pm on the 7th the doctor decided that the baby was getting tired and to be certain of healthy baby and healthy mother it was far better to short cut the affair and do the operation. As the specialist in the ante-natal clinic the previous week had told the students, when holding a post-mortem over my body, that day never hesitate to do a cesarean section on an elderly mother if her labour was prolonged. I was not in the least surprised or discouraged when the Dr. came and told me they were taking this course. I just said 'Good, because I want to be alive at the end and I want my baby' within ten minutes I was flat out and knew no more till 10 pm. (The baby was born at 8:40 pm) When I heard sister saying to my husband outside the room where I was 'I don't think she knows she has a son: We didn't tell her.'

The treatment and care in the _____ Hospital I found first class I enjoyed ward life—I was there two weeks and got home two days ago feeling (and I'm told looking) extremely well. I never got weak or sick as I was got up the morning on the first day. The baby was 7 lbs 8 oz when he left the hospital. He's a slow putter on and for the first eight or nine days I had little milk. They weren't sure if I could feed him entirely. However as I grew fitter it came and I [now] have an adequate supply which I hope will last till he's due to be weaned. As I'm placid, contented and very happy to have a son I expect it will continue to flow. The baby has taken to home life like a duck to water.

In many ways I'm sorry I didn't have the full experience of birth but being older I think it better to have my baby safe and sound. As things are at the moment tho's. . . I don't want an only child I hope I can and so does my husband—I really wanted five or six but I married too late for that. . . .

Yours sincerely,

4 October 1949

Dear Mrs.,

Thank you very much for your long and interesting letter. I feel the only remark I can make is that 'All is well that ends well.' I am so glad you were in first class hands so that all eventualities could be met in a successful manner.

I am so pleased to hear the nice things that you have had to say about the _____ Hospital. It is a magnificent place and is run by men of the best type.

All good wishes to yourself and your family.

Yours sincerely,
Grantly Dick Read, M.A., M.D., Cantab.

Correspondence 51

January 2, 1951
California

Dear Dr. Read,

I have finished reading Childbirth Without Fear. I would like very much to have my early-in May baby by your method. I am 40 years old. I think by re-reading parts of the book and trying very hard I could 'get' the technique.

Dare I do this with the following history?

Oct. 1941—10 lb. boy still born. Case of prolapsed cord. When he discovered the situation my doctor performed a 'version' pulling the baby out feet first. The shoulders were broad. The wall between the vagina and rectum was torn full length. A year later Doctor told me that during this long process he hadn't thought I'd pull through. At birth the babe had been dead about 7 hours.

Dec. 1942—Twins, boy and girl, 7 lbs and 6 3/4 lbs, born by Cesarean Section. Doctor was afraid of a normal delivery because he was afraid the large repair job of 14 months before wouldn't hold.

June 1947—Boy—9 1/2 lbs—born by Cesarean Section. This time Doctor would have permitted a natural birth but several nurse friends said that in a hard labor the old uterine scar might rupture. Doctor had told me that the first time my muscles 'hadn't worked at all,' so this time I was afraid. During this third hospitalization one of the nurses told me, however, that prolapsed cord cases are always slow.

So that is it! I really have a great desire to have this baby normally, I think partly because the first time I woke up feeling that there was no baby and asked twice before I was told (and feared to ask a half dozen other times). I've wakened from both Cesareans with the same dread. I went into that first labor very thrilled and without much fear because two good friends had described the birth of their babies as wonderful spiritual experiences.

These are my assets:

1. I am always wonderfully well during pregnancy. No morning sickness or anything to bother. The only thing now (and there was this in my last pregnancy) is an occasional long pain after a hard sneeze or a sudden twisting movement. I imagine this means adhesions. Would they bother?

CMAC:PP/GDR/D.111

2. I'm active. I plan to teach school till the end of February. There's forty five minutes tap-dancing every afternoon which I haven't given up yet.

3. Both surface scars healed beautifully at the time of the second Cesarean. Doctor 'couldn't find' the first scar on the uterus. He's a skillful surgeon, and a skillful obstetrician. He's slow to use gas. Lots of women say 'too slow.'

4. I think my uterus is pretty tough stuff. The first time it wasn't torn at all with all the strain of the version and high forceps delivery.

5. I believe I'd be a good subject for relaxing. I love to 'float' in bed when I first lie down, and in swimming it's quite a lark to lie in the water indefinitely and almost sleep, with just an occasional kick to keep my legs from dragging. Last night I criticized my relaxation. Found it wasn't complete in the back and abdomen. Would that come with practice? My habit is abdominal breathing rather than diaphragm breathing. Would that make abdominal relaxation more difficult?

This is a spur-of-the-moment letter. I'll probably laugh at myself for writing it. But if you receive it, I hope you'll write me a note telling me what you think. Please! I'm anxious to see Doctor _____ and tell him I've read your book. Wonder what he'll say!

Sincerely,

9th February 1951

Dear Mrs.,

Thank you very much for sending me the record of your experiences in childbirth. I wish I were in a position to give you a more dogmatic reply to the questions that you put to me.

As I read your letter I am impressed with one or two facts. First, you do make very large children, and that is always a great strain upon a Cesarean scar, even though it is lower uterine segment operation and even though it was perfectly performed. If you did manage to develop a smaller child, and if your doctor was present during the whole of your labor prepared for an immediate Cesarean operation, you might still have a chance of a natural birth. Unfortunately, however, we can never predict whether a Cesarean scar will behave itself during the last six weeks of pregnancy. I have delivered a woman of an 8 lbs. 13 ozs. baby after two classic Cesarean operations, but she was under my vigilant eye for the last six weeks of pregnancy. She was only 32 years of age, and from the moment that her labor began I sat with her and had the operating theater fully prepared to perform a Cesarean section at a moment's notice. I also had an anesthetist and an assistant on the spot. This was an exceptional case. I am sending to you by seamail a reprint from the Lancet, on page 14 of which you will read a note on women who presented themselves to me demanding natural labors—some idea of the many points that must be taken into consideration will be clear to you.

You have written to me upon a very interesting subject, and there are still many gynecologists who believe that once a Cesarean section always a Cesarean section; they consider that the risks I take in this matter are quite unjustifiable. Up to date, however, the Gods have been kind to me and not one of the cases selected as suitable for physiological labor after one or two Cesarean sections has gone wrong. I dare not make any statement, however, that will be of help to you personally because I am not in a position to judge all the circumstances.

My best wishes,

Yours sincerely,
Grantly Dick Read, M.A., M.D., Cantab.

Correspondence 52

27 August 1954
London

Dear Dr. Read,

At 35 I am expecting my first baby at the end of November. Can you please help me to find somewhere to go where I can have my baby by your methods.

Fortunately I have read your books, and they make the whole process of having a baby seem so beautiful that I found myself actually looking forward to the event, but I am very disappointed to find that the clinic in my district has not adopted your system, and therefore has no relaxation or exercises. Also at the Maternity Home attached, the matron, while not being actually against relaxation, is not particularly in favour of it.

I have consulted my own Doctor on this problem and he has been very helpful in trying to find out if I can have the baby privately by your system, but he cannot find anything that would cost less than £70. As my husband is just an ordinary working man this is more than we can afford, but we could spend up to £35.

I do so hope you might know someone to whom I could go, because I want very much to have my baby naturally, and to find that it is a wonderful experience, than be put off from having another one for ever as has been the case with my sister.

Yours faithfully,

21 September 1954

Dear Mrs.,

I am so sorry your letter has not been answered before, but I have been away.

I usually recommend the people who write to me to get in touch with Dr. _____ of _____ Street, and put everything clearly and frankly to him, how much they can afford, where they would like to have their babies and whether he can assist them to go somewhere where my methods are being carried out efficiently.

And mind you, you must be careful Mrs. _____, at some of these

CMAC:PP/GDR/D.32

places you find there is a good deal that is not done adequately. _____
Hospital is worth going to because it is as near as anywhere to doing
the job properly. I don't know whether you could possibly have your
baby down at _____ where there is a Dr. _____ who is, I understand,
quite good at carrying out my procedures. He worked with me for a
short time, and you could have your baby there under the National
Health Service if you wished to do so. His address is _____.

    I am sorry I cannot be of more definite help to you but these sugges-
tions may ultimately be of some service.

Yours sincerely,
Grantly Dick Read, M.A., M.D., Cantab.

Correspondence 53

10 October 1956
London

Dear Dr. Grantly Dick Read,

I was so very terribly moved by your broadcast this afternoon, that I must let you know of my own experience.

When I became pregnant after six months of marriage I told my mother, who was horrified and told me I would never survive it and ought to have an abortion, on medical grounds. I had never had any illness apart from childhood epidemics, so of course I ignored her reactions and reported to the hospital monthly, felt very fit and worked till the very night my daughter was born (as a secretary). However I think deep down her words must have frightened me, for I had the most ghastly time, although only five hours labour, with 'twilight' and eventually some anesthetic for I never knew the baby was born.

My daughter is now 13 and I am 40. She has always longed for brothers and sisters, asking me almost daily for years, but there, I felt I couldn't do it again. Of course this has affected my life and that of my family enormously, and of course my relations with my husband. If I could be sure of an easy childbirth, after all these years, I would try, but what do you think? It is so tragic for my little girl.

Yours truly,

P.S. May I thank you for all the work you have done for womankind all over the world!

28 November 1956

Dear Mrs.,

I am almost invariably humiliated when I look at the date upon the letters as they come to the top of this enormous pile which always waits to be answered. I was most grateful to read what you wrote to me, and it is of course for women who have suffered as you have suffered, not only of the body but of the mind, that my work is possibly more espe-

CMAC:PP/GDR/D.49

cially offered. Perhaps one of the greatest tragedies of the civilized peoples is that their minds are very rarely prepared for the most wonderful experience of their lives.

How frequently I have had to say, it is with the mind that babies are born of the body is so largely subjected to the mental processes which govern it. I can only offer you this consolation, that with adequate preparation another child born with all the joy that you know can be obtained. A very considerable number of women of forty and over have been to me to ask if they are too old to have another baby, and the consolation is this. I find that the statistical results of the births of babies at that age are extremely good and with a little girl of 13, you could rejuvenate not only your whole home and the atmosphere of the home, but at the same time you could bring into her life something which would make her understand the tremendous privilege of being a woman.

I expect you will understand and appreciate that I believe the greatest gift of a woman is mother-love and certainly it is the greatest power in the world today. There is nothing that crosses so easily the bridge that stretches over the gulf between human and spiritual life. I cannot urge you to take any step, but I have seen so much happiness from the late born babies and so much health that I certainly cannot advise you not to consider seriously with your husband all the pros and cons of another child.

My best wishes,

Yours sincerely,
Grantly Dick Read, M.A., M.D., Cantab.

ATTEMPTED SELF-ABORTION

Correspondence 54

December 7, 1951
New Jersey

Dear Dr. Read,

I do not know if you will ever receive this letter. I can only hope and pray that you will because I know myself to be a perfect example of the uneducated and ignorant American female regarding natural childbirth.

I am a young woman of twenty three who grew up in a closely guarded convent school, in which sex, or anything pertaining even remotely to a woman's true function in life was never discussed except by whispers among the students and then rarely because they knew more than I. When my first menstruation period arrived I was ill and scared silly because I had not even been informed that this phenomenon would eventually occur. Upon leaving this cloister at the age of eighteen I still knew next to nothing about the facts of life.

I am telling you all these things because I wish you to understand how really ignorant I was—so much so, that it is truly incredible. For one thing only am I grateful—I had also never had an opportunity to hear these 'old wives tales' of the horrors of child birth which I have been hearing during the past few months. Otherwise, I fear that they would have been so firmly imbedded into my mind as to be practically indestructible.

I am now entering my eighth month of pregnancy. Oh, if only I had heard of you earlier how many weary hours of heartbreak and uncertainty might have been avoided! Since living here on the [Army] Post I have had an opportunity of meeting many young women of my own age who have already had children and I have at the risk of making myself an infernal pest, asked many questions. 'What is it like, having a child? Did your baby kick very much? Mine does very strongly at times and then for no apparent reason, he will be quiet for several days. Why is this? It worries me so much at times and since it is probably a very normal thing I hate to bother the doctor with such questions. Is it very

CMAC:PP/GDR/D.105

painful—the actual birth? How can such a small opening expand sufficiently to permit passage of a child's head?'

Oh, so many interminable questions doctor? And the answers are
always too vague. Actually what they all boil down to eventually is 'Believe me, it is more than worth the torture!' Now I ask you, what was I
to believe? If you only knew how many nights I have cried myself to
sleep! This was another phenomenon that worried me greatly. Tears
came so easily—I who had never permitted events to upset me—I was
gradually becoming a real cry-baby! I had foolish fancies that my husband did not love me any more. I found myself watching his every action and word and interpreting an ulterior motive behind each. I convinced myself that he was totally indifferent to the baby that is coming
and proceeded to nag him about everything.

I now know that all these strange tricks of my imagination originated
at one fundamental source—fear—fear of the unknown. And then I
had the good fortune of meeting a young Englishwoman whose husband is attached to the Air Corp on this Post. One day she casually
mentioned that she was re-reading your book 'Childbirth Without Fear.'
She is in the sixth month of pregnancy and it is her second child. Like a
dying man grasps a straw in the hope of survival I casually inquired if I
might read the book when she had finished. You see, I had reached the
stage where I was too embarrassed to ask any more questions about
child birth because I had been snubbed so many times, and by this time
was hypersensitive to mine [sic] own ignorance of which I was so thoroughly ashamed.

I have just finished reading your book and oh, how very right and
true it is! I can testify to that with my whole heart from my own little
experience of pregnancy. I suffered no vomiting or upsets at the onset
of pregnancy and why? You have answered that! I did not know I was
pregnant and when realization gradually dawned and was affirmed by
a doctor my only reaction at first was anger. Why did it have to happen
to me! I didn't want a child to tie me down. I was young and happy and
very much in love with my husband. I was afraid to tell him because I
did not know how he would react. We had so very little. Without consulting anyone I became determined to get rid of this child because I
was convinced that it would be only a millstone about our necks. My
doctor had given me all the do's and don'ts' [sic] of pregnancy by word
and also in a little pamphlet. I proceeded to do all of the donts' [sic] with
more vigor than I had thought myself capable of. I built a rock garden,
dragging every stone and pound of loam up over the hill in a wheelbar-
row. Even my husband remonstrated that I must not work so hard or I
would kill myself—and he didn't even know I was pregnant!

By the time the garden was finished I was convinced that overwork was not going to do any good. Gradually, I became resigned to the thought of having a baby and that resignation gradually developed into joy and wonder so that I could no longer keep the good news to myself. I told my husband one night. He took me in his arms and held me very close for a while without saying anything. Finally he looked down into my face with the look of an old and worn man and said, 'We must start to save money and prepare for it right away.' I know now his anxiety for me—my health—for I have always been frail as you will know when I tell you that I stand 4'11" and weigh normally only 76 pounds. But on seeing the hunted look in his eyes while he forced that twisted smile to his lips I thought 'I am killing him. Now he will worry so about where the money is to come from. It isn't fair! I am making him old before his time, making him bear too heavy a load of responsibility!' Surely you can understand then why I began to hate and despise the child I carried in my womb with more violence than I had believed possible. As the financial strings tightened so did my bitterness deepen toward its cause.

My one salvation at this time was my deep sense of religion. Thank God, for that! Through the hate and fear came the realization that I had no right to blame this defenseless creature which God had placed under my protection. When he began to stir in my womb I experienced fullness of heart—and a fierce desire to protect which I suppose is the origin of mother love. I know now, deep in my heart that I love this child I carry with my whole soul, and that the only compensation I can ever accept after he leaves my womb in emptiness, is the feel of his body in my arms. The longing to hold him there, to feel him flesh and blood, and truly mine grows hour by hour and day by day.

I want to bear my child naturally without drugs for only then will I feel that he is truly part of me and I am determined that nothing will stand in my way this time.

I write this to let you know how profoundly your book has touched me, and after my child is born I shall make it my business to see that no young girl is left in ignorance of the true facts. Never will I hesitate to answer any question they put to me. I will study hard that I may know the truth and be able to pass that truth on to others as clearly and as logically as God gives me words.

Thank you again most sincerely for your wonderful book. I only wish more people could read it and realize its significance. In my own small way I will try to help others know the truth.

Sincerely,

28th December 1951

Dear Mrs.,

I have received your letter and in reasonable quick time. It is a most interesting document, not only because of the vivid manner in which you have written it, but because of the portrayal of a psychological experience, which to a greater or lesser degree has frequently been brought to my notice.

When I wrote a small pamphlet called 'Motherhood in the Post-War World,' published I think for 6d by Heinemanns, I had in mind to a large extent such people as yourself. I advocated the early training of girls, and even went further by suggesting that before the age of 18, the senior classes of all schools should be brought into direct contact with the domestic duties of young mothers, and should have a knowledge of the care of babies, which would supplement a sound instruction of that most beautiful of all physiological functions, the conception and birth of a child.

How much pain and distress you would have been spared had it been your lot to receive such an education. I notice in your letter that you wrote when you were in your eighth month of pregnancy. It is possible, therefore, that this letter will not arrive until after your baby is born; if that is so, I sincerely hope that all went well with you, and that you were able, with the close assistance of those in attendance upon you, to follow out the procedures which my years of experience have told me to be so worthwhile. If your child has not yet arrived, may I adjure to patience, courage and self-control, realizing that if you can allow your uterus to give your child without interference or anxiety, and you will experience the most wonderful event that it is within the lot of a young girl to know. I shall be pleased to hear from you when you have time to write to me how your labor goes. My best wishes for a very happy and successful New Year in your new role of mother and wife.

Yours sincerely,
Grantly Dick Read, M.A., M.D., Cantab.

There was no further correspondence between them.

DEATH OF DOWN'S SYNDROME CHILD

Correspondence 55

June 7, 1948
Indiana

Dear Dr. Read,

I suppose you receive many letters from women who have read your books; I doubt if any are as grateful as I. Because of that gratitude, I am prompted to tell you about my labor, the results, and my present state of mind.

I had such a wonderful time. . . .

. . . my pains started at 7:30 A.M. at about fifteen minute intervals. For a while I just gloried in them. At 10:00 I called my doctor. Since I had an hour's drive in ice and snow he told me to come right in. After that I washed and dried my hair. I tell you that to demonstrate the agony I was enduring. I then drove myself to the hospital while my father timed my pains and took care of my mother. My husband, being a doctor, was already there.

The rest of the day was spent playing bridge with Dr. _____ and friends.

My son was not born until thirty hours after the first pains. So that I could sleep, I was given one hundred milligrams of Demerol which was worn off long before I reached the second stage.

The delivery, Dr. Read, was the greatest experience of my life. I would awaken from the amnesiac sleep you speak of to 'bear down,' I bothered everyone with questions. 'Was that the membranes?' etc.

After one great effort, I felt such tremendous relief. I propped myself up and asked if the head had been born. It was, and I was told if I'd lie down and push again, I'd be a mother. I did and I was. My only regret is that I again fell asleep and missed my baby's cry.

Now why do I bore you with a story you've been told countless times? I looked at a baby I thought was beautiful. But I have not the critical eye of a physician. Six days later Dr. _____ told me our son was Mongoloid, and our only course was to hospitalize him.

I carried him home for baptism on that day and returned him to the hospital where he passed away two months later.

CMAC:PP/GDR/D.106

You speak in your book of women who dread a second pregnancy because of the torture of the first. Imagine me if I had those memories and no child as a reward. I have you to thank that Infant B's birth is not an ugly memory of pain or drugged sleep.

As it is, six hours after my child was born I was walking around. You probably don't approve [of] that—my attending doctor didn't. My post-partum, until I received that news, was delightful.

Now, less than four months later, I have sadness but also the knowledge that I am again pregnant. No one approves of that either, but the peace of mind it brings assures me my body will stay healthy.

So Dr. Read, forgive this imposition on the time of a busy man. Indirectly, you've helped me overcome a situation which might have prevented the birth of many children I hope to have. For myself and Dr. [her husband] I had to thank you.

Sincerely,

7 August 1940

Dear Mrs.,

I was pleased to receive your letter, as indeed I always am when my teaching has been of service to those whom I have not the pleasure of knowing personally. I was indeed grieved to read that you had that great tragedy, for not long before I received your letter two girls whom I was looking after had a similar unhappy experience. I am quite sure, however, that you are right in your attitude. Those who can be tried in the fire of misfortune and emerge with sound phylosophy [sic] have a streak of true greatness. I have no doubt that this will be applicable to your motherhood, which indeed you deserve to enjoy.

When and if I revisit America, as I hope to next year, it would give me great pleasure to meet you and Dr. [the husband], although Indiana is a little off the beaten track.

I can do no more than send you my best wishes, and remind you of the three great virtues which I preach to those who invite my attentions. They are not only applicable in labor, but throughout motherhood—patience, self-control, and the ability to work hard cheerfully.

Yours sincerely,
Grantly Dick Read, M.A., M.D., Cantab.

EPISIOTOMY

Correspondence 56

June 22, 1952
New York

Dear Dr. Read:

Both my husband and I have read your book chapter by chapter in preparation for our first baby.

When I made my first visit to our doctor and we talked about natural childbirth he told me that he had taken a special course in this method and had already delivered ten babies easily and without anesthesia.

However he advised that since this is my first child that a slight incision be made at the time when the baby's head is about to be born for the following reasons: 1) to avoid possible tearing of muscular walls and to prevent later muscular weakness in the abdomen and 2) to avoid an oversized uterus afterwards which he says will diminish the mutual enjoyment of intercourse since the uterus is too large to give full enjoyment to either partner.

I am in good health and my measurements are good, he has told me. I asked if it was not possible to follow your exercises both before and after birth to avoid the possibility of tearing and the result of an overly enlarged uterus. He replied that his experience has been that it is better to make this incision with a first child and to avoid the above and that secondly it is not possible to exercise enough to return the uterus and muscles to the proper condition once they have been overly stretched.

Since I want to have the baby naturally but do not wish to have the results he mentions as being possible I have wondered if this was prejudice on his part or whether it is true in the case of a woman giving birth for the first time.

Both my husband and I would very much appreciate hearing from you.

Sincerely yours,

CMAC:PP/GDR/D.111

13 August 1952

Dear Mrs.,

I am sorry that your letter has taken both so long to arrive and also such a long time for me to answer, but my correspondence gets on top of me some times.

I appreciate your letter and it raises a question which is very difficult to answer for no two women are alike. There are those who have a very small and rigid outlet at the vulva and such cases, as the head advances, the obstetrician has to judge whether it will dilate sufficiently to allow the head to pass without any rupture. For my own part I very rarely do the episiotomies, that is to say, the cut at the opening. On the other hand I do fairly frequently have a small snick of the mucus membrane just inside which requires one relatively painless stitch to draw it up into shape again.

The question of the muscular weakness or the oversize of the vagina afterwards giving rise to troubles with intercourse. There seems to me to be a very poor argument; if you do the exercising of the muscles of the pelvis this can be overcome so easily and in the majority of cases there is absolutely no difference except possibly a considerable improvement in coitus after a child has been born.

Of course, in America there is a considerable [opinion] towards doing episiotomies on everyone as there is towards giving anesthetics to everybody, but I don't think that anyone who has had a baby as you describe need be bothered with those rather hypo-overscientific aspects towards childbirth.

My kind regards, I hope all will go well with you,

Yours sincerely,
Grantly Dick Read, M.A., M.D., Cantab.

HUSBANDS AND CHILDBIRTH

Husband Delivered the Child

Correspondence 57

November 30, 1952
New York

Dear Dr. Read,
  Exactly five months and five days ago, my husband delivered our
second child. It was not by accident, nor is my husband a doctor. Having read every word of three books written by you, I believe you might
like to hear our story.
  [My husband] and I first read about 'Natural Childbirth' shortly before we were married in 1950, when I was 17 and he 19. (An article
about the Yale University School of Medicine in New Haven, Conn.,
appeared in 'Life' magazine.) We decided that we wanted our future
children to be born the way God intended them. Unfortunately, this is
almost an impossibility in our society today. . . .
  It wasn't until my sixth month of pregnancy that we finally located
(or so we thought) a doctor who referred to himself as a 'Natural Childbirth' doctor. This specialist was quite a distance from our home but
we figured the time, effort, and money involved would be well worth
it. However, it turned out that the obstetrician we had chosen was an
advocate of your teachings in theory only. Outside of a book of exercises and a monthly check-up, no other pre-natal care was given. Consequently, I did the preparatory exercises and followed a sensible diet
on my own, looking forward to the day when I would see my first child
born. My husband was allowed to stay with me during labor and in the
delivery room. However neither the doctor nor hospital made other
provisions for a natural birth. Consequently, when I entered the delivery room I was treated as though I were unconscious and within minutes I was screaming for ether. (It's interesting to note that I had been
relaxed and happy in the labor room with my husband for twelve hours
preceding my trip to the delivery room.) As a result, I missed seeing the
birth of my first child by a few minutes. I won't bother with details, but
needless to say, the methods employed by the obstetrician certainly
were not natural. The post-natal care at this expensive hospital was

CMAC:PP/GDR/D.106

terrible, and my husband and I finally succeeded in procuring my re-
lease two and one-half days after the baby's birth. (I should like to mention here that even though I hadn't had a natural birth I was walking
about a few hours after my son was born. I attribute this to the fact
that I was so relaxed throughout those twelve hours of labor.)

At this point my husband and I wondered what other doctors of less
importance, and hospitals *less* expensive, would be like. We assumed
they would be no better, if not worse, especially since natural childbirth
was almost un-heard of.

And so my first child was not even three days old when [my hus-
band] and I decided to have another one soon, and that my husband
would deliver it. I was very frustrated, wanting to prove to myself that
I could have a natural birth if I had a fair chance.

Perhaps you think we were a little radical planning to deliver our
own child but I should like to explain why we knew we would be successful.

First of all, both my husband and I were bright students in school.
As a matter of fact I won a scholarship to New York University which I
attended for one year. So feeling that we were equipped with a certain
amount of intelligence and common sense, we proceeded to plan my
second pregnancy. (Before our first son was one year old.)

I purchased your three books: 'Childbirth Without Fear', 'Introduction to Motherhood', and 'Birth of a Child'. It didn't take me long to
read thru them from cover to cover, as once started I couldn't put them
down. I kept to a sensible and nourishing diet and of course carried out
my exercises. This comes easily as I have always been unusually ath-
letic. Also, I have large bone structure and excellent posture.

Besides knowing that I was both mentally and physically equipped
to bear a child naturally, [my husband] and I decided we would try to
carry out the same procedure a doctor follows during periodic visits.
For instance I noted my increases in weight and took my own urine-
sugar analysis tests. Three weeks before the baby was due we had a
chiropractor friend of ours x-ray the baby. It was in excellent position
as we had expected. (I should like to mention that I have an elaborate
chart which contains information from the first time I menstruated. I
call it my 'Cycle History.' Consequently I was only three days off in
figuring the birth date of my first child. The doctor was two weeks off.)

I hope I have adequately explained why we felt that God-willing, we
would have a perfectly natural, uncomplicated birth. A couple of weeks
before I expected the baby, I sterilized some sheets and other things
which I thought we would need.

When the great day came we were all ready. My labor lasted six hours. At one time I almost lost control but [my husband] gave me much encouragement and the head was soon born. I hardly felt that, but I shall never forget the feeling of the entire body being born. [My husband] immediately handed me the baby and I awoke from my amnesiac state as though I had been struck by lightning. The baby surprised us by being so large (8 lbs. 4 oz.) as I had gained less than fifteen pounds. The placenta practically lept out and there was no tear of the perineum, and practically no blood.

I was walking about soon after the baby's birth and on the beach in a bathing suit the following day. Before he was five days old I was in complete charge of the house and my nineteen month old "terror." By the way, the new baby is the most contented child ever born. He never wakes us at night and is always smiling.

We have only one regret: [My husband] had cleaned our cameras with alcohol, meaning to have a picture of the baby's birth, but he was so excited he forgot all about it. Perhaps it's just as well. No photo could ever describe that moment.

We do have a picture of the entire family taken when the baby was two hours old. I have taken the liberty of enclosing a reprint. Please excuse the lack of clothing. The baby was born during the hottest part of the day on one of the hottest days in June.

My husband and I are trying our best to spread your theory on Natural Childbirth. . . . Perhaps, some day it will be the usual practice among doctors and hospitals. I hope so. It's surprising how few of our acquaintances believe in natural birth. They think that having successfully delivered our own child we are either mad, lucky, ignorant, or that I am extraordinarily healthy. There are a few exceptions.

Sincerely,

19th January, 1953

Dear Mrs.,

I am very pleased that you should have written to me so fully about your experiences in childbirth, and it was a kindly thought that you should send me the delightful picture of the family quartet.

It is people like yourselfs [sic] who can be so much good in this world by removing the fear of childbirth and by emphasizing what tremendous happiness it brings to husband and wife if carried out according to the natural design.

I am interested to read that many of your acquaintances think you are either mad or in some other way a bit odd. This was very common twenty years ago, but today, with the very rapid spread of this essentially commonsense approach to motherhood, it is not heard so frequently. You can be sure that in a few years they will alter their views.

My best wishes to you and again thank you for having written to me.

Yours sincerely,

Grantly Dick Read, M.A., M.D., Cantab.

HUSBANDS AND CHILDBIRTH

Husband Requesting Advice

Correspondence 58

20 November 1954
Palmers Green

Dear Dr. Read,

I wonder if you would help us. The problem in its simplest form is, where, within the means of ordinary people, are the principles laid down in your book, 'Childbirth Without Fear,' practiced?

We had our first baby six months ago after waiting three years for it. We are longing for more, but my wife is dreading the prospect of future confinements after her last experience. The delivery would doubtless go down in the records as normal, and our baby girl is strong and thoroughly healthy, but the fact remains that my wife, who is highly strung, suffered hell. And there is no doubt in the minds of either of us that the trouble was largely if not entirely that she was harassed by the midwives. We know that some of the midwives at the particular hospital are extremely good but the element of uncertainty—they might have left, be on leave or off duty—is unsatisfactory. My wife has a natural tendency to worry, in spite of being exceptionally intelligent, and always thought she would prefer to have her baby in hospital because of facilities in emergencies; now she thinks a home confinement would be best (because of the peace) but this might be unsatisfactory because she is Rh [negative].

My wife read 'Introduction to Motherhood' and the one already mentioned during her pregnancy and was convinced by your arguments. It is interesting to note, since it confirms what you say in 'Childbirth without Fear,' the events leading up to the delivery of the baby:

Contractions began at 2:45 a.m. We got up at 3:45 and left for the hospital at 5:30 after my wife had insisted on tidying the house, leaving her clothes and the babies' [sic] things ready for her return and having a bath. At the hospital she remembered all she had read and remained perfectly composed all during the first stage of labour. At 9:30 a.m. she was fully dilated and was taken into the labour ward where the trouble began. Commands came one after another with monotonous regularity—

CMAC:PP/GDR/D.30

'Right now, PUSH'
'But I don't feel the urge'
'Oh, well don't push yet.' Pause
'Right NOW push.'

Three people seemed to be dashing round, in and out, and after a very short time my wife felt thoroughly mixed up, and actually thought 'Oh, it's all gone wrong, if only I could begin again.' At one point a midwife even said 'Come on, *hurry up*, other people are waiting!' And in the ensuing hours of orders and pummellings my wife said 'Oh shut up' (much to her subsequent surprise). The baby eventually arrived at 6 p.m. the same day.

If you could tell us where we could be sure of the right clinical conditions and psychological atmosphere we would be extremely grateful. I realise you are not an enquiry bureau and that you have a great deal to do with your time; I shall therefore be more than pleased with even a couple of lines in reply. Please forgive my presumption in writing to you; only the tremendous importance of the matter to us, and the knowledge that you have put so much effort into solving similar problems, prompts me to do so.

Yours faithfully,

20 November 1954

Dear Mr.,

I appreciate you having written to me and I do hope I can be of some help to you. Unfortunately your letter is one of such a very large number who have the same sad story to tell, that a girl has learnt her job, she has got the courage and she is blessed with the ability to have her child as women were obviously intended to have them, and then has it ultimately rather messed up by the attendants in the labour ward. It is such a shame.

But we are getting on, and as you know I have been struggling at this for forty years now, and at last it is being received generally and there are a large number of hospitals where you can get very much more sympathetic understanding treatment than your wife appeared to receive when her last baby was born.

You didn't tell me what hospital you had been to, so it makes it a little difficult for me to know how to advise you, but I certainly think you would get very much better treatment today at _____ Hospital under Professor _____'s staff. Of course, if you have got a doctor locally and you can get a good midwife who really understands her work, and your wife has her baby at home, probably she would be very much happier. The only catch in that is being a rhesus negative and I do think it would be wise for her to be under the care of a first class hospital staff, in case she happened to be one of the four per cent of rhesus negative women who tend to develop what we call antibodies, because that needs a little extra care for the baby, as you know after it is born. But that should introduce no difficulty at all providing she is in good hands.

Try _____ Hospital and mention my name to Professor _____ when you write, and tell him exactly what you have told me about this last birth and why you want to go there. I think you will find he will be of the greatest possible help to you.

Yours sincerely,
Grantly Dick Read, M.A., M.D. Cantab.

HUSBANDS AND CHILDBIRTH

Homosexual Husband

Correspondence 59

23 January 1956
Suffolk

Dear Dr. Read,

As soon as my husband knew that I was going to have a baby he bought me your wonderful book, 'Introduction to Motherhood,' and that was six months ago, now I am able to thank you for teaching me in a simple way the things that happen to my body and when I am having my baby, in fact I am so looking forward to having my baby that I feel like a child who has just been told that a wonderful party is soon going to take place. I have followed your exercises and I can honestly say that no-one would know that I was expecting a baby if I didn't tell them. There is however one thing that is bothering my husband and myself and that is that I can't make my doctor of the Nursing Home see how badly I want my husband to be with me through the actual birth. Until recently my husband has been a homosexual letting others do this horrible act to him but not returning it. He is illegitimate and consequently had a very disturbed childhood. I married and loved him knowing full well the difficulties and moods I would encounter and I am wonderfully happy to say that love has won through. He now gives me his full affection but I am so frightened that his will not stay so if he can't share the most wonderful moment of my life—the birth of our baby. Please can you help me I am sure the nursing home would listen to your influence. My doctor is wonderful but although he agrees with most things you say he cannot see why the husband at the birth of the first. . .is so necessary as complications are likely to arise but yet he says my husband could be there at the birth of the second, third, etc. babies! I did not know of anyone whose influence I could safely rely on except you so please forgive me for writing to you a very busy man.

Yours faithfully,

CMAC:PP/GDR/D.51

28 February 1956

Dear Mrs.,

Thank you very much for your letter and I am so sorry it hasn't been answered before. I think I agree with you almost one hundred percent in the questions as to whether your husband should be present at the birth of your first baby or not. You didn't say by the way when it is likely to arrive.

If he is interested himself fully in the subject and has read with you 'Introduction to Motherhood' so that you can understand together what goes on, so that he himself can know how he can be of help to you and not be present only to satisfy his own curiosity, then I must say I would favor his presence.

On the other hand, as I say quite clearly in the third edition of 'Childbirth Without Fear,' that husbands should not be there unless they can be of help to their wives. By that I mean offer her a companionable sense of security and give to her the pride of his presence which helps so many girls to have their babies nicely. If he is not perfectly willing to play his part, then he should be asked to go outside. So far as having a first baby goes, I think he can help a lot particularly when you may get to a stage when you may have some backache for a short time. If there is any difficulty, which is very unlikely, in my opinion then the doctor can certainly ask him to go outside and wait.

That is the method I used in my own practice before I retired, and I suppose about thirty percent of husbands were present for some part of the labour and ten or twelve percent of them were there all the time. I think this number would have been very much higher had the babies been delivered in their homes and not in hospitals. Hospital regulations make it a little difficult sometimes and of course we have to sympathize with the authorities in those institutions as well.

Your case does, however, seem to have a rather special indication for, as you say, this complete experience together but finally I must tell you I cannot possibly give you one hundred percent advice because I don't know your husband and that is so necessary from my point of view.

Another thing is that I do ask you in particular to realize how much having a child demands your courage and self-control. It is not a picnic and it is not for a girl to have her first baby easy, it is hard work, it is the examination of her womanhood but no woman who really keeps her self-control and understanding has anything whatever to be afraid of except herself, and if she gives herself to the laws of nature and allows

them to have her baby, can look forward to having no unbearable discomfort or difficulty.

My best wishes to you,

Yours sincerely,
Grantly Dick Read, M.A., M.D., Cantab.

MENSTRUATION

Correspondence 60

October 28, 1952
New Jersey

Dear Dr. Grantly Dick Read,

I have recently read your book 'Childbirth Without Fear' and think it is wonderful. And I have taken the liberty to write you about my daughter who suffers from menstruation pains.

I would like to know is there any book or article you could suggest her reading on the subject of 'menstruation without fear,' or any relaxing method that would help these pains to disappear, or anything else you would suggest.

This is a great worry to me and I would be very grateful for anything you would suggest.

I hope you will forgive my boldness in writing you.

My daughter has had the minor operation called dilation but although the pains are some less she still suffers badly.

Thanking you so much for any help you would give.

Very sincerely yours,

13 December 1952

Dear Mrs.,

I see that you are in New Jersey, and I strongly recommend that you make the journey, which I hope will not be too long to see Dr. _____.
He is a friend of mine whose work I admire and whose ability is unquestioned. You will appreciate my difficulty in not seeing your daughter, or knowing the type of menstrual pains she has, or indeed what her age is. It is a very wide subject and the general causes of this distressing complaint are:

1. Psychological
2. Hormone system of the body not being well balanced and
3. Some organic inflammation of the urethra and urinary bladder.

CMAC:PP/GDR/D.100

I have not known simple dilation of the cervix of the uterus successful in many cases unless psychological treatment has also been applied. If you can get from any medical library, 'Psychosomatic Gynaecology' by Kroger and Freed, you will find a lot of very sensible reading upon painful menstruation. You might also be able to find a copy of the English medical journal called 'The Lancet' (10th February 1951) in which there is a paper by myself on Ureteric Dysmenorrhoea. I have had great success with this treatment in a large number of cases which otherwise were not possible to cure.

I cannot give you very full advice, but I do like to feel that I am of help to anyone who comes to me, but I assure you the wisest course would be to go and see Dr. _____ and talk the matter over with him, even going back to the years before your daughter started her periods, and I hope you will be able to find some relief for this poor child.

My best wishes,

Yours sincerely,
Grantly Dick Read, M.A., M.D., Cantab.

MISCARRIAGE

Correspondence 61

28 September 1948
Michigan

Grantly Dick Read, M.D.
c/o Harper and Brothers
London, England
Dear Sir:

This letter is addressed to Dr. Read with the hope and trust that as author of 'Childbirth Without Fear,' he would find it possible to answer these questions, which arose from an effort to apply his theories of fear and pain.

Upon learning I was pregnant, it was comforting to discover that my doctor and the well-known hospital of which he was a staff member, believed in Dr. Read's book—but! Time, they told me, did not permit them to practice it. Incidentally, it was at this time I 'discovered' Dr. Read's book. I was in a book shop and came across the name 'Read, Grantly Dick' and the association of the name with a much criticized article in a magazine caused me to verify author and so I came to read 'Childbirth Without Fear' and then to re-read it with conviction and faith, faith that this time I would carry my pregnancy through successfully.

With a past medical history of three miscarriages, I began my fourth pregnancy at 36 with the again-familiar and repetitive symptom of 'spotting.' With this exception: I stopped spotting after 23 days, although I took no medication and did not stay in bed, since all previous miscarriages occurred even while confined to bed.

On August 19 I miscarried at 4 1/2 months after a visit to the doctor showed I had started to dilate.

My history should include the fact that I am about 10% deficient in thyroid, even though I took thyroid from age 16 to 32 (for irregular periods) *without any beneficial results.* My periods averaged 4 a year until more recently they began averaging 8 a year, 6 weeks apart, and sometimes skipping a month. The improvement in regulating periods seemed to follow an operation for ovarian cysts, following the third miscarriage.

CMAC:PP/GDR/D.105

With the other pregnancies, much care was taken and vitamin B and E, Progesterone, and thyroid; and yet miscarriages occurred. During this pregnancy no medication was taken or prescribed. The doctor had suggested some thyroid on my second visit, but it was postponed because of my trouble with rapid pulse. I blame myself for this postponement. Each pregnancy was carried one month more than the previous one. If Dr. Read was appalled at unprogressive ideas held on childbirth, I am distressed at the 'mystery' surrounding miscarriages and their use. Is there any hope for me to have a baby? If there is a serious omission in Dr. Read's book, it is this: why aren't miscarriages discussed? Normal women with uncomplicated deliveries will not read the book. I've talked with them—they're not interested and smile at [the] phrase 'painless childbirth.' Now they even imply some sort of justification for their mistrust simply because my pregnancy ended unhappily. And this question goes unanswered: why do women tensed with fear and women who break every rule of health still manage to give birth to healthy normal babies? I saw in the labor room three screaming women, (one with four fibroid tumors) delivered of healthy babies.

There is one point on which no conflict exists—fear causes pain and even illness as doctors are beginning to acknowledge.

Very truly yours,

4 November 1948

Dear Mrs.,

Thank you for your letter which was a very sad manuscript. Of course I must make it clear to you that the book I published in America, 'Childbirth Without Fear,' neither discusses abnormal obstetrics or miscarriages. It is entirely confined to normal and natural childbirth. The woman who has frequent miscarriages suffers most distressing disappointment. The causes are innumerable. They may be a fault in chemistry, in the position of the uterus or even in the emotional attitude of the woman towards childbearing, but in your case I feel I must give you the results of a wide investigation which we have made in this country recently, which points to the possibility that recurrent miscarriages are due in quite a high percentage of cases to a low grade of spermatozoon produced by the husband. In many cases recently a full investigation of the husband's semen has revealed subfertility. When this has been corrected the shape and size of the male fertilizing agent improved, by one of the many means which scientists have at their disposal today, firm and healthy pregnancies have resulted and full term children born.

You have asked me to discuss this matter with you and I do so on the assumption that any suggestions I make to you will be used only as suggestions and possibilities and not as a diagnosis of the cause of your misfortunes. I am willing to be of this service to you because of the confidence that infuses the letter that you sent me, because it is a demand for help which as a physician I believe should not be denied those who make serious enquiries. You must of course show this letter to your husband and make him realize that it contains no aspersion upon his manhood, his physical ability or his mental acuity. We have not yet aspired to the powers of the Almighty but so far as we have been allowed to understand these mysteries we are willing to impart understanding to others.

Yours sincerely,
Grantly Dick Read, M.A., M.D., Cantab.

RELIGION AND NATURAL CHILDBIRTH

Correspondence 62

12 December 1955
South Devon

Dear Dr. Read,

Our fourth child is now one day old and I felt I wanted to write to you and thank you for the part you played through your book, 'Revelation of Childbirth,' in giving me four wonderful experiences and four healthy, happy children.

I read your book when I was expecting my first infant, and was deeply impressed by your outlook on childbirth and your clear explanation of this natural process. Although unable to attend clinic, (we live in the country), I tried to carry out the exercises and relaxation as you described and was fortunate in having a doctor who agreed with your methods.

All our babies were born at home and for the last three the doctor has been a mere spectator—nevertheless an encouraging one—the nurse and I getting on with the job. You would doubtless not have thought me an ideal patient, as I did experience a lot of discomfort at the end of the first stage, and succumbed to the temptation to have some pethedin (only half a dose though, and not any for the third child). After that, when I could settle down to doing some work, I had absolutely *no* desire for any sort of analgesic. Though gas and air was always offered me. I feel this was almost entirely due to reading your book, with its wonderful dispelling of fear and ignorance. I wish every Mother would read it! The sense of utter fulfillment and well being on seeing and feeling one's baby born and holding it immediately after birth defies any description. The worst of it is, it increases one's already swollen head! Incidentally, I never experienced the feeling that I was going to burst or split, which you mention in your book as a common sensation—perhaps because of your reassurance that this will not in fact occur. Our babies were not small either—the one born yesterday weighed 8 lbs 12 oz.

There is one thing I would like to add out of my experience and that is the wonderful way in which prayer, (not just messages for help!) can assist in relaxation. I have tried, especially during the last pregnancy, to make the daily period of relaxation one of prayer and with the result

CMAC:PP/GDR/D.42

that one is not only physically relaxed but mentally and spiritually too. During this last confinement I found that to 'Let Go and Let God' was far easier and more effective than just to 'Let Go.' If ever you write another book will you bear witness to this? I know you must be a Christian because of the preface you wrote for the Guild of Health's Leaflet for pre- and post-natal Services of Blessings and Thanksgiving.

I have become more and more convinced during the last few years that to try to grow nearer to God through learning true prayer is the only hope for any of us in this present troubled world.

No answer is expected to this as you must receive hundreds of similar letters but please accept my gratitude for your enlightening book, which you may be sure I shall recommend to as many mothers-to-be as possible.

Yours sincerely,

15 December 1955

Dear Mrs.,

I have received your letter this morning and I am most grateful to you for writing so fully to me.

You say no answer is expected, but although I do receive hundreds indeed thousands of letters from mothers who have been happy in childbirth through this very natural approach, yours is one of especial value because you have mentioned so clearly an aspect which I am quite sure is of immense value.

The short, aphorism, 'Let Go and Let God,' is beautiful. A very popular woman's magazine has asked me to supply them with something which will stimulate their readers and to recognize the value of natural childbirth and what it can mean to mothers other than just having their babies comfortably. Providing I do not use your name or give any clue to the writer, do you think you would be good enough to allow me to offer this to her for her next issue. I know it would be of tremendous help to a very large number of mothers, which I am quite sure is as near your ambition as it is to mine.

Will you be kind enough to send me a postcard with either 'yes' or 'no' on it so that your family duties and Christmas preparations are not disturbed by writing letters.

May I wish you and yours every happiness at this time.

My best wishes,

Yours sincerely,
Grantly Dick Read, M.A., M.D., Cantab.

19 December 1955

Dear Dr. Read,

Thank you for your letter—I did appreciate your prompt reply. I should be only too pleased for you to use my letter in any way you think fit, provided as you say, there were no names mentioned! But there is one thing I must mention in fairness to you, and that is that phrase, 'Let Go and Let God,' is not, I regret, original. It is the title of a book, which I saw advertised in 'Church Illustrated' some months ago, (but which I have never read and cannot even remember the name of the author I'm afraid), and it stuck in my mind to such an extent that I found myself thinking of it repeatedly during the first stage contractions of my last labour. It was incredibly wonderful how God did take over when He was invited to.

I do hope that copyright difficulties will not prevent you from using this somewhat apt phrase in your article.

With all good wishes to you and your family for Christmas.

Yours sincerely,

30 December 1955

Dear Mrs.,

Thank you very much for your letter of December 19 and for the information with regard to the origin of the phrase, 'Let Go and Let God.' I do appreciate these details and I have written to the Rector at _____ about it. With my best wishes to you and your family for a very Happy New Year.

Yours sincerely,
Grantly Dick Read, M.A., M.D., Cantab.

UNMARRIED AND PREGNANT

Single Woman

Correspondence 63

18 September 1951
Herts

Dear Dr. Dick Read,

I am reading your book, 'Childbirth Without Fear,' because I am interested in practicing relaxation methods when I have my baby in December.

In the chapter on the Phenomena of Labour you say that a state of chronic mental tension is frequently the cause of minor ailments in pregnancy. I am in rather a difficult position regarding this 'mental tension.'

I am unmarried and the father of the baby is already married, and rather than cause any trouble or difficulty in his home by asking for maintenance I am bearing the cost myself. I feel, as I was selfish and thoughtless enough to let my emotions overcome my common sense, that I shouldn't make others suffer for my mistakes.

When the baby started I'm afraid I tried several pills and remedies for this but it seemed the only way. I then told my parents, who were wonderful, and have arranged that I should go into a home of reeducated girls to have the baby—and then have it adopted.

This is my problem. I got a job as a mother's help right away from home, and once away and able to think matters out I find I very much want the baby. I've always wanted a family—since I was quite small, and think what a wonderful thing this is to be actually carrying a real baby. The sordid side of matters, which was much the atmosphere at home, has disappeared.

As soon as I realized that the baby really *had* to be—then I tried to take every care and give him the opportunity of developing under happy and contented circumstances.

I am a trained nurse and last year went in for midwifery, but gave it up after only 3 months in the hospital in which I was training was grossly understaffed and I felt that to carry on with such cruelty to the patients, which it was—as we never had time to be *real* nurses, kindness

CMAC:PP/GDR/D.39

and thoughtfulness were merely in theory—practice it was just running, shouting at screaming frightened women and the whole thrill of delivering a baby quietly and peacefully in a calm atmosphere was out of the question.

I felt so much then, before I had read your book, that childbirth should not be accompanied by this turmoil and pain, and so rather than do something with which I could not agree, I gave it up.

Do you think that under the circumstances I can expect to carry out relaxation wholly successfully? I want the baby so very much, but don't know that if I kept him it might not be giving him every chance in the future as he would have with two parents. It is such a problem to decide.

My parents will not think of keeping the baby, but I can support him fairly well, I think, with my training behind me. I am 23 years old. I feel that unless I can settle this problem I might not be able to relax properly. I am practicing your exercises, but wonder, from my small experience of maternity work whether the hospital to which I go to actually have the baby will leave me alone to do things peacefully, or will they disturb the whole procedure by being interfering. Do you think that one can shut out such interference, or would the strain on the emotions be too great to relax?

I do hope you don't mind my writing to you like this, you must have so many patients with so many problems. If fees are required for your advice, please may I have pre-notice of your charges?

I feel so ashamed of bringing a baby into the world without a father, but I am determined to do my best to see that the baby has every chance that a child with a normal home would have. I am looking forward to the actual confinement very much, as I am so sure that childbirth should be natural and according to your theory.

If you should reply to this letter will you please address the letter to MRS., as I am having to be 'married' for the good of those girls who may follow me in my present job, and who are in the same position as myself. This organization with which I am in contact is very wonderful and so helpful, finding jobs for the girls until 6 weeks before confinement and keeping one in the home until 6 weeks afterwards. I am so very grateful for all they have done for me. The utter dispair one has, when faced with a problem like this, all alone, is so much relieved by these wonderful people.

My other problem is probably I think one of the signs, or outcomes of mental tension, though I have relieved that greatly. It is severe pain in the muscle of the left thigh joint, almost a burning pain, which is marked when I lie on my back with knees bent. If I get into this position it takes a good deal of maneuvering to get up again. Hence at times I find the exercise for, leg raising alternately and lowering slowly, rather difficult, also the exercise for stretching the pelvis.

I am taking the Ministry of Food Vitamin Tablets and orange juice and also Vit B 3 mg. t.d.s. I have chronic constipation, which I treat with Parrafin and Phenothalein Emubion. The doctor I am registered with here is very kind and interested, but can give no answer to the painful hip muscles, which I would like to deal with if possible, as I am sure it is not natural to suffer this pain.

I do apologize of presuming to write to you, but hope you can advise me, if not I shall quite understand as you of course can not answer everyone's problems.

Thanking you.

Yours faithfully,

CONFIDENTIAL
21 September 1951

Dear Mrs.,

I have read your letter and it leaves me with a sense of admiration that there are still women with your strong and sensible instinct towards that which is right for the children they bear.

I have attended some hundreds who have found themselves in a position similar to yours, but not always have they been so fortunate in their own choice of parents. The fact that your father and mother have exhibited the good and human qualities you describe is an asset beyond value.

I strongly suggest to you that for the next year or two your life revolves about the infant that is yours, before and after its birth. Children require warmth and comfort and dependence upon the mothers who bear them.

Forty years behind the scenes of personal life has made me critical of those who would accuse. I have quoted many times a short saying which you will recognize, and there is probably nothing in the life of Christ more applicable to modern society. 'He that is without sin among you, let him cast a stone at her.'

My advice to you is, as it has been to scores of others. Maintain the integrity of your child, do not part with it. It needs *you*. You can pose, if it is necessary to palliate the so-called society in which you will live, as a widow, or anything you wish. You must expect to receive chastisement, especially from those who have never known love, or had the opportunity of bearing a child. As soon as you can, take a job as a trained nurse, and live somewhere away from your people and your friends in a home where your baby can be cared for whilst you are earning your living during the day. It will not be long before a girl with your outlook and courage will find a man who falls in love with her for what she is, and not for the foolish errors that she might have made, if they can be called that.

I do not condone lack of control, in fact I condemn it. If a person wishes to walk in the mud and gets into trouble, I do not put my foot on his neck and push him under. I prefer to pull him out, put him under the garden hose, kick him where he deserves it and tell him not to do it again.

If your parents do not want you to keep this child, I suggest that you ask them whether their family pride, which is quite justifiable, is in any way comparable to the sin of taking a mother from her child. You certainly have no reason to get overwrought and tense with your situation. Lift up your chin and realize that because your indiscretion becomes obvious it is incomparably less harmful to those amongst whom you live, than the malice of evil tongues, the scourge of jealousy and the vice of a life of deception. Besides who is your judge?

It reads as though you are taking care of yourself perfectly well, and your painful hip is probably due to the position of the baby. If it is the left thigh that troubles you persistently, relax during rest periods on the right side of your body and overcome the constipation which you complain of, by taking TAXOL. One after lunch and one at night.

I have written to you as I would have talked to you, had you come to my consulting room. The only difference is that I shall not have the pleasure of looking after you.

Yours sincerely,
Grantly Dick Read, M.A., M.D., Cantab.

UNMARRIED AND PREGNANT

Divorced Woman

Correspondence 64

15 January 1956
Sussex

Dear Dr. Dick Read,

I know that you will receive so many letters after your article in the 'Graphic' that I'm afraid mine may get lost in the avalanche, but I feel I must write to you.

I am having my first baby in June. My age is 36. The circumstances are difficult as I am awaiting a divorce (which, thank God, I now know will be through in time for me to remarry), and in addition I have serious money problems to face.

I mistakenly chose a woman doctor and wishing to be honest told her a little of my problems. She's a good, genuine woman but has completely got things wrong. Is loading me with sympathetic advice, including how to have my little baby adopted, etc., etc., and not one word of medical advice or suggestion that I attend a clinic. I admit I am a little scared, as I had a nasty internal operation for fibroids that gave me an example of abdominal pain, and I have a T.B. history and a miscarriage to my credit. But, doctor, I do want this little mite and to prepare for it as well I possibly can. I work funny hours and also must disguise my pregnancy as long as possible but I feel I can't go on in this blind ignorance and mixture of fear and joy between which I seem to alternate.

My sister runs a baby home and is Mothercraft trained, and she and her patients have such faith in you that I feel I must appeal to you for help and advice.

I cannot afford very heavy fees, but if I could possibly see and talk with you at least once I am sure I could gain confidence and peace of mind.

Yours sincerely,

CMAC:PP/GDR/D.47

24 January 1956

Dear Mrs.,

I was pleased to get your letter, because I am always happy to lend a hand if I can but I have retired now and don't know what to say. . . .

If I may offer speculative advice, I don't think I should be worried about anything. When all is said and done, let's look at the thing quite fairly. You have got that privilege which the large majority of women envy you for and it is a very great gift to become pregnant. I say that with all commonsense.

Secondly, you are in a bit of a domestic jam by waiting for a divorce. You don't say whether you are being divorced or you are divorcing your husband, but I don't think that matters much, if it is the step you have decided to take, get on with it and face the fact quite obviously and the future quite plainly.

I naturally cannot make any comments on your doctor's attitude towards this, but if you are a little scared of it because of internal operations, T.B. history, miscarriages and the what-not, ask yourself why? So many people look right past commonsense into trouble when it isn't really there at all.

What I strongly suggest you do is go to every hospital and nursing home . . . . and try and discover someone who is running an antenatal class to assist you to get properly prepared. Get hold of my books one of them, 'Antenatal Illustrated,' 'Introduction to Motherhood,' or 'Childbirth Without Fear' (best of all if you can afford 10/d) and see what you can do. There is not the slightest reason why you should have any more trouble than hundreds of thousands of women all over the world today who are having their babies naturally and so happily. I am not going to tell you that you won't have to work hard and on the specific day you may get some aches and pains, but nothing bad enough for you to need major assistance or interferences.

I couldn't agree with you more when you write that your fear is in blind ignorance. Very well, in that case get hold of that book and you will find why fear is due to ignorance and why joy is so justified to any woman in the world, divorced, single, married or anything else you like, who is about to become a mother.

Take that tip from me. Go and find an antenatal school, go and find a hospital or nursing home where you can get someone to look after you in the way you want and I am perfectly certain you will write to me in the very far distant future and say 'I had the most wonderful baby, and I am going to stick to it—there is not question of anyone else having it.'

My best wishes to you and write to me again if I can be of any help.

Yours sincerely,

Grantly Dick Read, M.A., M.D., Cantab.

Glossary of Medical Terms

Accoucheur - birth attendant

Analgesia - pain relief that does not cause the patient to lose consciousness or fall asleep

Anesthesia - lack of awareness of pain with or without lose of consciousness

Antenatal - the British term for prenatal

Birth Canal - passageway through which the baby is born; the uterine opening and vagina

Cesarean Birth (C-Section) - surgical delivery of the fetus by incisions through the abdominal and uterine walls

Cervix - the lower, narrower end of the uterus which the baby passes through to enter the vagina

Chloroform - a sweetish, colorless, volatile liquid; administered by inhalation

Confinement - the time period of labor and delivery; childbirth

Contractions - rhythmic tightening of the muscles in the upper part of the uterus during labor

Coombs' Test - mixing antihuman serum, produced in rabbits, with the erythro-cytes of the infant; clumping indicates the presence of antibodies coated on the erytyhrocytes

Demerol - a trademark for a narcotic drug that relieves pain (meperidine); pre-scription analgesic used in labor and delivery

Dilatation and Curettage (D & C) - widening of the opening to the uterus (cer-vix) and scraping the lining (endometrium) of the uterus. A D&C is done to diagnose diseases of the uterus, to correct heavy vaginal bleeding, or to empty the uterus of substances from conception (as after a miscarriage or in an abortion).

Dilatation - gradual opening of the cervix

Enteritis - inflammation in the lining of the bowels, often the small intes- tine; causes include bacteria, viruses, and some functional disorders

Episiotomy - small cut made in the tissues (perineum) at the opening of the vagina to enlarge the passageway

Ether - inhaled as a general anesthetic; it has an irritating, strong oder and is highly flammable and explosive; often causes nausea and vomiting after surgery

Forceps - instrument used to deliver a baby; specifically they assist in the birth of the fetal head and vary in length, shape and way of action

Gas and air - analgesic inhaled and administered by the patient

Hematoma - pooling of blood that escaped from the vessels and became trapped in the tissues of the skin or in an organ

Hysterectomy - an operation which removes the uterus; performed either through the abdominal wall or through the vagina

Induction of Labor - an obstetric procedure in which labor is begun artificially by rupturing the fetal membranes or giving a drug. It is done because of the condition of the fetus or the mother requires it or for the convenience of the mother or the obstetrician

Instrument Birth - see forceps

Labor - rhythmical contractions of the uterine muscles that open the cervix and expel the baby, membrances, and placenta

Membranes - "bag of waters;" a sac of thin membrances in which the baby floats within the uterus during pregnancy

Midwife - a person who helps women in childbirth

Nembutal - a trademark for a barbiturate (pentobarbital) used as a sedative

Nitrous Oxide - a gas used as an anesthetic

Nursing home - place where women gave birth in Britain

Parturient - describing a woman in labor

Pelvis - basin-shaped ring of bones at the bottom of the trunk of the body which supports the spine and rest on the legs

Perineum - tissues between the anus and the vagina

Phenolphthalein laxative - a laxative that acts on the wall of the bowel; given to treat long-term constipation and to prevent straining

Placenta - sponge like organ attached to the uterine wall of the mother and by the umbilical cord to the baby; the baby receives its nourishment and expels its wastes by means of the placenta

Postnatal - after the baby is born

Prenatal - before birth

Primipara a woman who has given birth to one, live infant

Puerperium - period of time following birth until the pelvic organs return to the nonpregnant condition

Rh factor - a substance (antigen) in the red blood cells of most people. A person with the factor is Rh+ (Rh positive). A person lacking the factor is Rh- (Rh negative). If an Rh- person receives Rh+ blood, red blood cells are destroyed and anemia occurs. An Rh+ fetus may be exposed to antibodies to the factor made in the Rh-mother's blood. Red cell destruction occurs and if untreated, a fatal condition results. Transfusion, blood typings, and crossmatching depend on Rh+ and ABO blood group labeling. The Rh factor was first found in the blood of a species of the rhesus (Rh) monkey. It is in the red cells of 85% of people.

Scientific Childbirth - childbirth in the hospital, with drugs and instruments

Spina bifida - a nerve tube defect present at birth that results in a gap in the bone that surrounds the spinal cord

Uterus - organ in the female pelvis in which a fetus can develop; the womb

Vagina - passage from the cervix to the vulva

Vulva - external female genitals, composed of the inner and outer folds of tissue (labia minora, labia majora), clitoris, and vaginal opening

Books by Grantly Dick-Read

Books Published in England:

Natural Childbirth, William Heinemann, 1933
Revelation of Childbirth, William Heinemann, 1942
Motherhood in the Post-War World, William Heinemann, 1943
Birth of a Child, William Heinemann, 1947
Introduction to Motherhood, William Heinemann, 1950
Antenatal Illustrated, William Heinemann, 1955
No Time for Fear, William Heinemann, 1958

Books Published in the United States:

Childbirth Without Fear, Harper & Brothers, 1944
Birth of a Child, Vanguard Press, 1950
Introduction to Motherhood, Harper & Brothers, 1950
No Time for Fear, Harper & Brothers, 1950
Natural Childbirth Primer, Harper & Brothers, 1956

Bibliography

Primary Sources

Dick-Read, Grantly. Papers. Contemporary Medical Archives Centre. Wellcome Institute for the History of Medicine, London.

Secondary Sources

Books

Anderson, Karen. *Wartime Women: Sex Roles, Family Relations, and the Status of Women during World War II*. Westport, Ct.: Greenwood Press, 1981.

Arney, William Ray. *Power and the Profession of Obstetrics*. Chicago: University of Chicago Press, 1982.

Bock, Gisela, and Pat Thanes, eds. *Maternity and Gender Policies: Women and the Rise of the European Welfare States 1880–1950*. London: Routledge, 1991.

Bourne, Aleck. *A Doctor's Creed: The Memoirs of a Gynaecologist*. London: Gollancz, 1962.

Breines, Wini. *Young, White, and Miserable: Growing Up Female in the Fifties*. Boston: Beacon Press, 1992.

Davies, Margaret Llewelyn, ed. *Maternity: Letters from Working-Women*. New York: W. W. Norton, 1978, originally published London: G. Bell & Sons, 1915.

Dawson, Jill, ed. *Kisses on Paper*. Boston: Faber & Faber, 1995.

D'Emilio, John, and Estelle B. Freedman. *Intimate Matters: A History of Sexuality in America*. New York: Harper & Row, 1988.

Donnison, Jean. *Midwives and Medical Men: A History of the Struggle for the Control of Childbirth*. New York: Schocken Books, 1977.

Elshtain, Jean Bethke. *Public Man, Private Woman: Women in Political and Social Thought*. Oxford: Martin Robinson, 1981.

Fildes, Valerie A., Lara Marks, and Hilary Marland, eds. *Women and Children First: International Maternal and Infant Welfare 1870–1945*. London: Routledge, 1992.

Fox, Daniel M. *Health Policies, Health Politics: The British and American Experience, 1911–1965*. Princeton: Princeton University Press, 1986.

Harvey, Brett. *The Fifties: A Women's Oral History*. New York: Harper Collins, 1993.

Heron, Liz, ed. *Truth, Dare or Promise: Girls Growing Up in the Fifties*. London: Virago Press, 1985.

Honigsbaum, Frank. *The Division in British Medicine: A History of the Separation of General Practice from Hospital Care, 1911–1968*. London: Kogan Page, 1979.

Jalland, Patricia. *Women, Marriage, and Politics, 1860–1914*. Oxford: Oxford University Press, 1986.

Jordanova, Ludmilla. *Sexual Visions: Images of gender in Science and Medicine between the Eighteenth and Twentieth Centuries*. Madison, Wisc.: University of Wisconsin Press, 1989.

Ladd-Taylor, Molly. *Raising a Baby the Government Way: Mothers' Letters to the Children's Bureau, 1915–1932*. New Brunswick, N.J.: Rutgers University Press, 1986.

Leavitt, Judith Walzer. *Brought to Bed: Childbearing in America, 1750–1950*. Oxford: Oxford University Press, 1986.

———, ed. *Women and Health in America*. Madison, Wisc.: University of Wisconsin Press, 1984.

Lewis, Jane. *The Politics of Motherhood: Child and Maternal Welfare in England, 1900–1939*. London: Croom Helm, 1980.

———. *Women in Britain Since 1945*. Oxford: Basil Blackwell, 1992.

———, ed. *Labour and Love: Women's Experience of Home and Family, 1850–1940*. London: Basil Blackwell, 1986.

Loudon, Irvine. *Death in Childbirth: An International Study of Maternal Care and Maternal Mortality 1800–1950*. Oxford: Oxford University Press, 1992.

Martin, Emily. *The Woman in the Body: A Cultural Analysis of Reproduction*. Boston: Beacon Press, 1987.

May, Elaine Tyler. *Homeward Bound: American Families in the Cold War Era*. New York: Basic Books, 1988.

Mitchell, Juliet, and Ann Oakley, eds. *The Rights and Wrongs of Women*. Harmondsworth: Penguin, 1976.

Mitford, Jessica. *The American Way of Birth*. New York: Dutton, 1992.

Morantz-Sanchez, Regina Markell. *Sympathy and Science: Women Physicians in American Medicine*. Oxford: Oxford University Press, 1985.

Moscucci, Ornella. *The Science of Woman: Gynaecology and Gender in England, 1800–1929*. Cambridge: Cambridge University Press, 1990.

Oakley, Ann. *The Captured Womb: A History of the Medical Care of Pregnant Women*. Oxford: Basil Blackwell, 1984.

———. *Women Confined: Towards a Sociology of Childbirth*. New York: Schocken Books, 1980.

Pateman, Carole. *The Sexual Contract*. Stanford: Stanford University Press, 1988.

Poovey, Mary. *Uneven Developments: The Ideological Work of Gender in Mid-Victorian England*. Chicago: University of Chicago Press, 1988.

Rich, Adrienne. *Of Woman Born*. London: Virago Press, 1977.

Riley, Denise. *War in the Nursery*. London: Virago Press, 1983.

Roberts, Elizabeth. *A Woman's Place: An Oral History of Working-Class Women, 1890–1940*. Oxford: Basil Blackwell, 1984.

_____. *Women and Families: An Oral History, 1940–1970*. Oxford: Basil Blackwell, 1995.

Sandelowski, Margarete. *Pain, Pleasure, and American Childbirth: From the Twilight Sleep to the Read Method, 1914–1960*. Westport, Ct.: Greenwood Press, 1984.

Scott, Joan Wallach. *Gender and the Politics of History*. New York: Columbia University Press, 1988.

Shorter, Edward. *A History of Women's Bodies*. London: Allen Lane, 1983.

Showalter, Elizabeth. *The Female Malady: Women, Madness and English Culture, 1830–1980*. London: Virago Press, 1987.

Smith-Rosenberg, Carroll. *Disorderly Conduct: Visions of Gender in Victorian America*. New York: Alfred A. Knopf, 1985.

Stevens, Rosemary. *Medical Practice in Modern England: The Impact of Specialization and State Medicine*. New Haven: Yale University Press, 1966.

Towler, Jean, and Joan Bramall. *Midwives in History and Society*. London: Croom Helm, 1986.

Wertz, Richard C., and Dorothy C. Wertz. *Lying-In: A History of Childbirth in America*. New York: Schocken Books, 1979.

Wilson, Elizabeth. *Only Half-Way to Paradise: Women in Post-War Britain, 1945–68*. London: Tavistock, 1980.

_____. *Women and the Welfare State*. London: Tavistock, 1977.

Articles

Borinsky, Alicia. "No Body There: On the Politics of Interlocution." In *Writing the Female Voice: Essays on Epistolary Literature*, edited by Elizabeth C. Goldsmith, 245–56. Boston: Northeastern University Press, 1989.

Davin, Anna. "Imperialism and Motherhood." *History Workshop* 5 (1978): 9–65.

Fox-Genovese, Elizabeth, "Placing Women's History in History." *New Left Review* 133 (1982): 5–29.

Freedman, Estelle B. "'Uncontrolled Desires': The Response to the Sexual Psychopath, 1920–1960." *Journal of American History* 74 (1987): 83–106.

Goldsmith, Elizabeth C. "Authority, Authenticity, and the Publication of Letters by Women." In *Writing the Female Voice: Essays on Epistolary Literature*, edited by Elizabeth C. Goldsmith, 46–59. Boston: Northeastern University Press, 1989.

Jordanova, Ludmilla. "Natural Facts: A Historical Perspective on Science and Sexuality." In *Nature, Culture, and Gender*, edited by Carol P. MacCormack and Marilyn Strathern, 42–67. Cambridge: Cambridge University Press, 1980.

Kunzel, Regina. "Pulp Fiction and Problem Girls: Reading and Rewriting Single Pregnancy in the Postwar United States." *American Historical Review* 100 (1995): 1465–87.

Lomas, P. "An Interpretation of Modern Obstetric Practice." In *The Place of Birth: A Study of the Environment in Which Birth Takes Place with Special Reference to Home Confinements*, edited by S. Kitzinger and J.A. Davis. Oxford: Oxford University Press, 1978.

Morantz, Regina. "The Lady and Her Physician." In *Clio's Consciousness Raised: New Perspectives on the History of Women*, edited by Mary S. Hartman and Lois W. Banner, 38–51. New York: Harper Colophon Books, 1974.

Oakley, Ann. "A Case of Maternity: Paradigms of Women as Maternity Cases." *Signs* 4 (1979): 607–31.

———. "Normal Motherhood: An Exercise in Self-Control?" In *Controlling Women: The Normal and the Deviant*, edited by Bridget Hutter and Gillian Williams, 79–107. London: Croom Helm, 1981.

Pateman, Carole. "The Patriarchal Welfare State." In *Democracy and the Welfare State*, edited by Amy Gutman, 231–60. Princeton: Princeton University Press, 1988.

Scott, Joan Wallach. "Gender: A Useful Category of Historical Analysis." *American Historical Review* 91 (1986): 1053–75.

Scott, Karen. "'Io Catarina': Ecclesiastical Politics and Oral Culture in the Letters of Catherine of Siena." In *Dear Sister: Medieval Women and the Epistolary Genre*, edited by Karen Cherewatuk and Ulrike Wiethaus, 87–121. Philadelphia: University of Pennsylvania Press, 1993.

Solinger, Rickie. "'A Complete Disaster': Abortion and the Politics of Hospital Abortion Committees, 1950–1970." *Feminist Studies* 19 (1993): 241–68.

Watt, Diane. "'No Writing for Writing's Sake': The Language of Service and Household Rhetoric in the Letters of the Paston Women." In *Dear Sister: Medieval Women and the Epistolary Genre*, edited by Karen Cherewatuk and Ulrike Wiethaus, 122–38. Philadelphia: University of Pennsylvania Press, 1993.